Praise for *Mastering the Art of Letting Go of Emotional Pain & Toxic Relationships*

"*Mastering the Art of Letting Go of Emotional Pain & Toxic Relationships* is both practical and deeply empathetic—a true gem. Dr. Puryear creates a safe space where vulnerability is celebrated as strength, a message especially powerful for teenagers. The hands-on exercises, like writing rituals and boundary-setting, make the lessons tangible and transformative. With its holistic approach that touches on social pressures, relationships, and independence, this book is an invaluable resource for educators, mentors, and anyone seeking healthier emotional balance."

—Marie-Hélène Fasquel, Readers' Favorite

"What I loved most about *Mastering the Art of Letting Go of Emotional Pain & Toxic Relationships* was how it moved beyond theory to provide practical, easy-to-follow exercises I could apply in both personal and professional life. Dr. Puryear writes with honesty and depth, turning each chapter into a step toward healing and self-discovery. The journey felt intimate and transformative, bringing reflection, inspiration, and genuine growth. It's a heartfelt and enlightening guide I highly recommend to teens, young adults, parents, educators, and wellness professionals alike."

—Salina Coria, Readers' Favorite

"*Mastering the Art of Letting Go of Emotional Pain & Toxic Relationships* is a compassionate and transformative guide that helped me rediscover my strength and self-worth. Dr. Puryear beautifully blends practicality with empathy, showing that choosing yourself is an act of deep love. His thoughtful strategies, reflective exercises, and mindfulness practices make healing both accessible and personal. This book reminded me that pain does not define me and that resilience, self-awareness, and emotional intelligence can turn even the hardest moments into profound growth."

—Jessica Barbosa, Readers' Favorite

"*Mastering the Art of Letting Go of Emotional Pain & Toxic Relationships* is a truly empowering and compassionate guide that made me feel both capable and supported. Dr. Puryear's encouraging approach shows that real change is within reach, offering practical tools to release the past and build healthier relationships. His thoughtful guidance fosters trust, self-awareness, and emotional balance, leaving readers with the confidence that peace and freedom are not just possible—they're attainable through mindful, loving choices."

—Asher Syed, Readers' Favorite

"*Mastering the Art of Letting Go of Emotional Pain & Toxic Relationships* is an inspiring and educational guide that makes emotional healing practical and attainable. Dr. Puryear's thoughtful exercises and clear takeaways help readers internalize each lesson and apply it to daily life. By focusing on self-compassion, mindfulness, and empathy, the book offers a grounded approach to reducing stress and anxiety in a fast-paced, demanding world. It's a must-read for anyone feeling weighed down by expectations and ready to reclaim peace of mind."

—Pikasho Deka, Readers' Favorite

"Some of us have been through a revolution just to survive our upbringings, not to mention living in a world filled with corruption, abuse, and lies. It's the resilient who survive, and it's books like *Mastering the Art of Letting Go of Emotional Pain & Toxic Relationships* that give you the tools to not only survive the muck, but prevail and live joyfully no matter what you've been through. Read this book and follow the advice for resilience!"

—Angela Shelton, actress, screenwriter, film director, and producer

YOUR HEALING
STARTS
HERE

A 90-DAY GUIDED JOURNAL
FOR LETTING GO, REFLECTION
& EMOTIONAL RENEWAL

JEROME PURYEAR MD

*To every young individual who has experienced
the burden of any kind of pressure,
has endured unmerited suffering,
and is prepared to embrace personal tranquility.*

*This book serves as an homage to your fortitude
and a pathway to reclaiming your true self.*

HELP SPREAD THE WORD!

If this book has helped you *release an old hurt,*
set a healthy boundary, or simply *find*
a little more hope on a hard day,
I'd be so grateful if you'd leave a review on Amazon.

Scan the QR code below
to share your reflection.

Your words matter—your story can help someone else
begin their healing journey.

Each review helps others discover this work,
and reminds other teens and young adults
that they're *not alone* on the path to peace.

Your light inspires healing.
Your voice builds hope.
Keep honoring your journey—
I'm rooting for you every step of the way.

CONTENTS

Introduction
Your Journey to Letting Go

This journal is a compassionate companion on a transformative 90-day journey toward emotional liberation and personal empowerment. Carefully designed to guide you through a profound process over the course of 90 days, *Your Healing Starts Here: A 90-Day Guided Journal for Letting Go, Reflection & Emotional Renewal* provides the tools and space you need to acknowledge your pain, release the burden of toxic emotional weight, and courageously rebuild your inner strength.

Each day, you will find thoughtful reflections that encourage deep introspection, alongside letting-go practices tailored to help you shed what no longer serves you. Powerful mantras, breathwork exercises, and stress-relief poses are woven throughout, acting as anchors of positive affirmation and a source of unwavering encouragement as you navigate this healing path.

This guided journey will lead you gently through a process of profound self-discovery, inviting you to explore the depths of your inner landscape. It provides a safe haven for practicing forgiveness—both for yourself and others—a critical step in releasing past hurts and moving forward. Ultimately, this journal empowers you to become the conscious architect of your own peace, enabling you to build a life you love that truly reflects your deepest desires and well-being. Embrace this journey and discover the resilient, joyful person you are meant to be.

WHO THIS JOURNAL IS FOR

This journal is designed to accompany my self-help book *Mastering the Art of Letting Go of Emotional Pain & Toxic Relationships*. For the best experience, I recommend reading that book before starting this journal. But this journal can be used as a standalone self-reflection tool too.

Your Healing Starts Here: A 90-Day Guided Journal for Letting Go, Reflection & Emotional Renewal is for anyone who:

- Is ready to actively engage in a personal healing journey
- Feels weighed down by past pain, guilt, shame, or toxic patterns
- Wants to develop greater self-awareness and emotional resilience
- Seeks to build confidence and self-compassion
- Desires to set healthier boundaries in their relationships and life
- Wishes to cultivate gratitude, embrace joy, and create a positive vision for their future
- Is committed to personal growth and self-improvement

This journal is for people who are prepared to dedicate time and effort to their emotional well-being and are open to guided reflections and practical exercises to achieve lasting peace.

HOW TO USE THIS JOURNAL

This journal is structured as a 90-day guided experience, divided into 12 weekly themes. Here's what you'll find in the journal:

Self-Assessment

On the next page, you'll find a self-assessment. Before you begin journaling, complete this self-assessment and take a moment to honestly reflect on where you are right now. This is not a test; it's a snapshot of your current emotional landscape. Revisit these questions at the end of your 90-day journey to observe your growth.

Weekly Focus

Every week, you'll find a new mantra and a central burden to release. Begin each week by reading the introduction to grasp the theme, and conclude the week with stress-relief yoga poses and mindful breathing and meditation videos. You'll find more information about each yoga pose and breathwork exercises in the appendix of this journal.

Daily Engagement

Dedicate time each day (preferably morning and evening) to engage with the journal prompts.

MORNING INTENTION: SETTING THE TONE FOR YOUR DAY

Begin your day with a deliberate act of consciousness by setting a clear intention. An intention is more than just a goal; it's a statement about how you choose to show up, how you want to feel, and the quality of energy you want to embody throughout the coming hours. It serves as an anchor, a mindful compass guiding your decisions, reactions, and interactions.

How to set your intention:

1. Reflect and Connect: Before getting out of bed or during your morning routine, take a few quiet moments to check in with yourself. What do you need today? What area of your life requires your most positive energy?

2. Formulate a Statement: Create a concise, positive statement, usually starting with "I will . . ." or "I am . . ." For example:

- I will approach challenges today with patience and a clear mind.
- I am present and fully engaged in every moment.
- I will speak and act from a place of kindness.

3. Choose a Guiding Word: Select a single word that encapsulates your overall intention and desired emotional state for the day. This guiding word is a powerful, easily recallable mantra that you can return to when you feel yourself losing focus or becoming reactive. Examples include:

- Calm
- Focus
- Joy
- Openness
- Presence

By setting an intention and choosing a guiding word, you proactively take control of your emotional landscape, ensuring that your healing journey is not left to chance but is instead an active, day-by-day commitment.

TODAY'S LETTING-GO PRACTICE

Engage with the specific exercise designed for that day, which could involve writing, mindfulness, or a physical act.

EVENING REFLECTION

Conclude your day by reflecting on challenges, strengths, and gratitude.

MOODS AND ENERGY LEVELS

Record how you're feeling today.

Reflection on the Past 4 Weeks

Every four weeks, take a moment to reflect on the journey so far with four simple journal prompts.

Final Days: Integration and Moving Forward

The "Final Days" section (Days 85–90) encourages you to revisit key themes and integrate what you've learned into your ongoing life.

Certificate of Freedom

At the end of the journal pages, you'll find a Certificate of Freedom. Fill it out with your name and the date you complete this journal.

This Certificate of Freedom is a powerful step, a symbolic declaration that you are consciously choosing to release the past. However, true emotional freedom is a journey, not a destination. This certificate marks a significant beginning—a commitment to let go—but the ongoing work of reflection, healing, and emotional renewal is what will solidify and expand that freedom into every area of your life. It is the foundation upon which you will build your lasting inner peace.

Appendix

The appendix contains essential information to guide your journey, including:

- Breathe, Release, Restore: 7 Days to Emotional Healing and Inner Peace
- Yoga Poses
- Breathwork Exercises
- Meditation Resource: *Mindful Moments*

Please refer to these resources as needed throughout the journal.

YOU'RE READY TO BEGIN YOUR 90-DAY JOURNEY

Now that you know how to use this journal, you're ready to begin. As you go through this 90-day journey, please give yourself compassion. Be completely honest in your responses. This journal is for you, and there's no right or wrong way to feel. Approach your reflections with kindness and understanding toward yourself.

Healing is not linear. If you miss a day, simply pick up where you left off. The goal is progress, not perfection.

This isn't just a journal—it's your personal blueprint for transformation. Every page invites you to reconnect with your truth, honor your healing journey, and design a life that reflects your worth.

Your journey to peace, confidence, and freedom begins the moment you open these pages.

Don't just heal—thrive.

Before You Begin
A Self-Assessment

Take a moment to honestly reflect on where you are right now. This is not a test; it's a snapshot of your current emotional landscape.

Note: To complete this self-assessment, use the rating scale provided in the instructions below to evaluate each statement.

INSTRUCTIONS
Rate yourself on a scale of 1 to 5, where:

> 1 = Strongly Disagree
> 2 = Disagree
> 3 = Neutral
> 4 = Agree
> 5 = Strongly Agree

EMOTIONAL WELL-BEING SELF-ASSESSMENT

1. I feel strong enough to face difficult emotions.

2. I can identify situations or thoughts that trigger my pain.

3. I feel comfortable expressing my true feelings and needs.

4. I am able to forgive myself for past mistakes or perceived shortcomings.

5. I feel a sense of worthiness and self-acceptance.

6. I have clear boundaries that protect my energy.

7. I regularly experience feelings of gratitude.

8. I feel hopeful about my future and can envision positive change.

9. I allow myself to experience joy without guilt.

10. I feel equipped to handle setbacks and maintain my peace.

REFLECT ON YOUR SCORES

Which areas did you rate lowest? These might be key areas to focus on during your journaling journey.

Which areas did you rate highest? Acknowledge your existing strengths!

What is one feeling you hope to cultivate more of by the end of this journal?

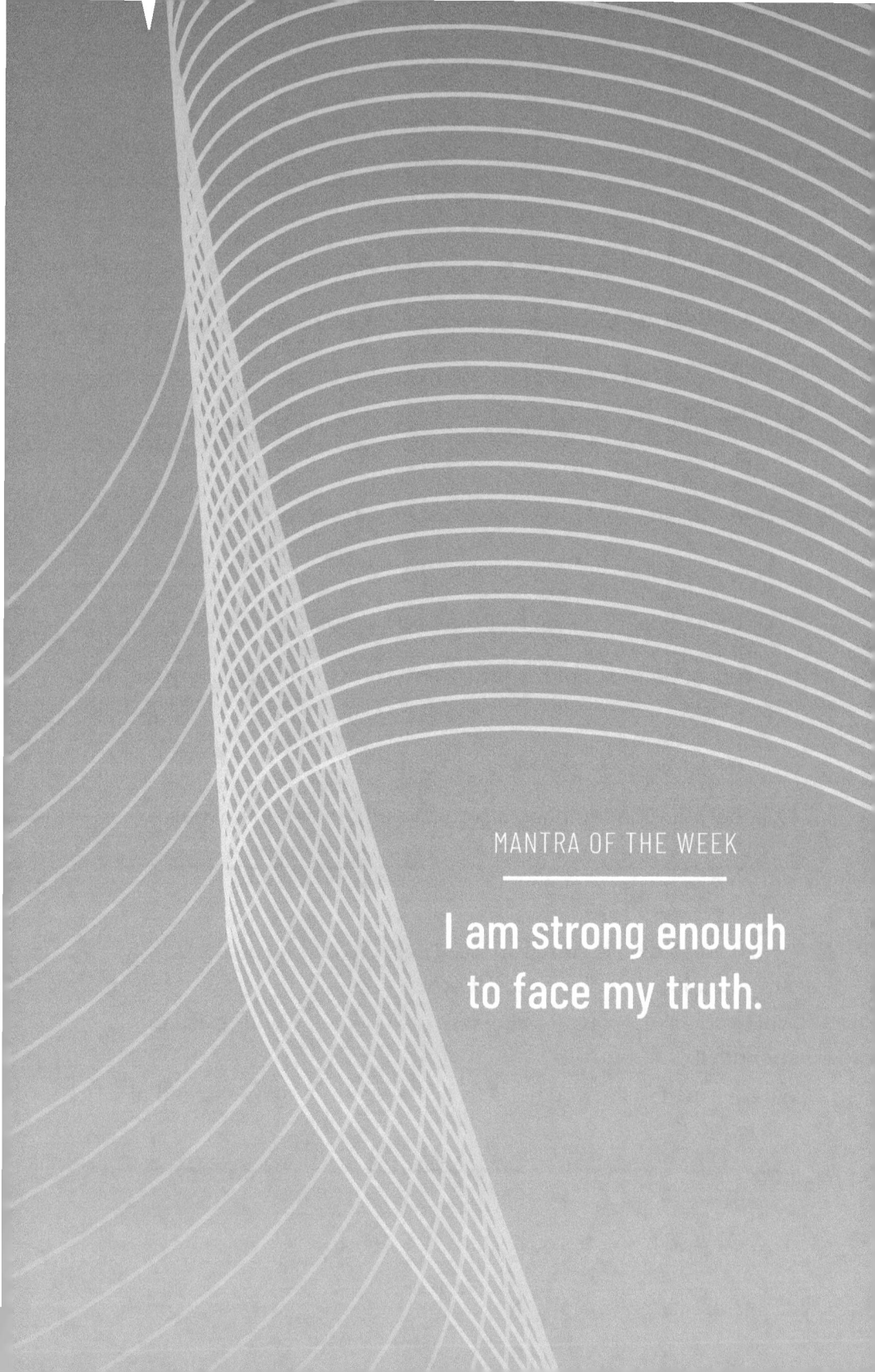

MANTRA OF THE WEEK

I am strong enough to face my truth.

Facing
the Pain

DAY 1

Morning Intention

Take a breath before you begin.

What am I noticing in myself this morning? (Thoughts, emotions, body sensations—anything that stands out.)

_____

_____

_____

Mood
How do you feel right now?
(Circle the one that represents how you feel.)

Energy Level
(Just notice—
this isn't about
motivation.)

How do I want to feel today?
(Write a word or phrase, or circle one.)

CALM • LIGHTER • STEADY • CONFIDENT
SAFE • FOCUSED • MYSELF

_____

_____

Today's Affirmation or Intention
(Keep it simple. One sentence is enough.)

_____

_____

*Today, I give myself permission
to take this one step at a time.*

Evening Reflection

*You made it through the day.
That matters.*

Mood
How did you feel overall today?

What challenged me today?
(Externally or internally—both count.)

_____

_____

_____

What helped me feel even a little stronger or lighter today? (Small things matter more than you think.)

_____

_____

_____

One thing I'm grateful for today:
(It can be about yourself, someone else, or a quiet moment.)

_____

_____

_____

Gentle Reminder: *If today felt heavy, that doesn't mean you failed. It means you showed up—and that's enough for today.*

TODAY'S LETTING-GO PRACTICE: Identify the Burden

Simply name the pain that feels heaviest. You don't need to fix it or analyze it yet. What is the one painful thought, memory, or relationship you want to focus on facing this week?

_____

_____

_____

_____

_____

_____

_____

DAY 2

Morning Intention

Take a breath before you begin.

What am I noticing in myself this morning? (Thoughts, emotions, body sensations—anything that stands out.)

_____

_____

_____

Mood
How do you feel right now?
(Circle the one that represents how you feel.)

Energy Level
(Just notice—this isn't about motivation.)

How do I want to feel today?
(Write a word or phrase, or circle one.)

CALM • LIGHTER • STEADY • CONFIDENT
SAFE • FOCUSED • MYSELF

_____

_____

Today's Affirmation or Intention
(Keep it simple. One sentence is enough.)

_____

_____

_____

Today, I give myself permission to take this one step at a time.

Evening Reflection

You made it through the day. That matters.

Mood
How did you feel overall today?

What challenged me today?
(Externally or internally—both count.)

_____

_____

_____

What helped me feel even a little stronger or lighter today? (Small things matter more than you think.)

_____

_____

_____

One thing I'm grateful for today:
(It can be about yourself, someone else, or a quiet moment.)

_____

_____

_____

Gentle Reminder: *If today felt heavy, that doesn't mean you failed. It means you showed up—and that's enough for today.*

TODAY'S LETTING-GO PRACTICE: Write to Understand

Describe how the pain you identified on Day 1 shows up in your daily life. How does it affect your mood, your energy, or your body? Write freely about the space it currently occupies.

_____

_____

_____

_____

_____

_____

_____

DAY 3

Morning Intention

Take a breath before you begin.

What am I noticing in myself this morning? (Thoughts, emotions, body sensations—anything that stands out.)

_____

_____

_____

Mood
How do you feel right now?
(Circle the one that represents how you feel.)

Energy Level
(Just notice—
this isn't about
motivation.)

How do I want to feel today?
(Write a word or phrase, or circle one.)

CALM • LIGHTER • STEADY • CONFIDENT
SAFE • FOCUSED • MYSELF

_____

_____

Today's Affirmation or Intention
(Keep it simple. One sentence is enough.)

_____

_____

_____

*Today, I give myself permission
to take this one step at a time.*

Evening Reflection

*You made it through the day.
That matters.*

Mood
How did you feel overall today?

What challenged me today?
(Externally or internally—both count.)

_____

_____

_____

What helped me feel even a little stronger or lighter today? (Small things matter more than you think.)

_____

_____

_____

One thing I'm grateful for today:
(It can be about yourself, someone else, or a quiet moment.)

_____

_____

_____

Gentle Reminder: *If today felt heavy, that doesn't mean you failed. It means you showed up—and that's enough for today.*

TODAY'S LETTING-GO PRACTICE: Act of Release

Find a quiet space and take three deep breaths. On each inhale, silently repeat, "I am strong enough." On each exhale, imagine you are releasing a small piece of the tension associated with your pain.

DAY 4

Morning Intention

Take a breath before you begin.

What am I noticing in myself this morning? (Thoughts, emotions, body sensations—anything that stands out.)

_____

_____

_____

Mood
How do you feel right now?
(Circle the one that represents how you feel.)

Energy Level
(Just notice—
this isn't about
motivation.)

How do I want to feel today?
(Write a word or phrase, or circle one.)

CALM • LIGHTER • STEADY • CONFIDENT
SAFE • FOCUSED • MYSELF

_____

_____

Today's Affirmation or Intention
(Keep it simple. One sentence is enough.)

_____

_____

_____

*Today, I give myself permission
to take this one step at a time.*

Evening Reflection

*You made it through the day.
That matters.*

Mood
How did you feel overall today?

What challenged me today?
(Externally or internally—both count.)

_____

_____

_____

What helped me feel even a little stronger or lighter today? (Small things matter more than you think.)

_____

_____

_____

One thing I'm grateful for today:
(It can be about yourself, someone else, or a quiet moment.)

_____

_____

_____

Gentle Reminder: *If today felt heavy, that doesn't mean you failed. It means you showed up—and that's enough for today.*

TODAY'S LETTING-GO PRACTICE: Mindful Detachment

For two minutes, focus only on the sounds around you. When your mind wanders to the painful feeling, gently acknowledge it and then guide your focus back to the sounds. The goal is to practice being the observer of your pain, not its prisoner.

DAY 5

Morning Intention

Take a breath before you begin.

What am I noticing in myself this morning? (Thoughts, emotions, body sensations—anything that stands out.)

_____

_____

_____

Mood
How do you feel right now?
(Circle the one that represents how you feel.)

Energy Level
(Just notice— this isn't about motivation.)

How do I want to feel today?
(Write a word or phrase, or circle one.)

CALM • LIGHTER • STEADY • CONFIDENT
SAFE • FOCUSED • MYSELF

_____

_____

Today's Affirmation or Intention
(Keep it simple. One sentence is enough.)

_____

_____

_____

Today, I give myself permission to take this one step at a time.

Evening Reflection

You made it through the day. That matters.

Mood
How did you feel overall today?

What challenged me today?
(Externally or internally—both count.)

_____

_____

_____

What helped me feel even a little stronger or lighter today? (Small things matter more than you think.)

_____

_____

_____

One thing I'm grateful for today:
(It can be about yourself, someone else, or a quiet moment.)

_____

_____

_____

Gentle Reminder: *If today felt heavy, that doesn't mean you failed. It means you showed up—and that's enough for today.*

TODAY'S LETTING-GO PRACTICE:
Reclaim Your Peace (Boundaries)

What is one small boundary you can set today to protect your energy from this pain? It could be declining to discuss a topic, limiting time on social media, or giving yourself permission to say "no" to one small thing.

_____

_____

_____

_____

_____

_____

_____

DAY 6

Morning Intention

Take a breath before you begin.

What am I noticing in myself this morning? (Thoughts, emotions, body sensations—anything that stands out.)

_____

_____

_____

Mood
How do you feel right now?
(Circle the one that represents how you feel.)

Energy Level
(Just notice—this isn't about motivation.)

How do I want to feel today?
(Write a word or phrase, or circle one.)

CALM • LIGHTER • STEADY • CONFIDENT
SAFE • FOCUSED • MYSELF

_____

_____

Today's Affirmation or Intention
(Keep it simple. One sentence is enough.)

_____

_____

_____

Today, I give myself permission to take this one step at a time.

Evening Reflection

You made it through the day. That matters.

Mood
How did you feel overall today?

What challenged me today?
(Externally or internally—both count.)

_____

_____

_____

What helped me feel even a little stronger or lighter today? (Small things matter more than you think.)

_____

_____

_____

One thing I'm grateful for today:
(It can be about yourself, someone else, or a quiet moment.)

_____

_____

_____

Gentle Reminder: *If today felt heavy, that doesn't mean you failed. It means you showed up—and that's enough for today.*

TODAY'S LETTING-GO PRACTICE: Express and Externalize

Draw a simple outline of a body. Using colors or scribbles, mark the places in the body where you feel the stress, sadness, or anger connected to your pain. Give the feeling a shape and color.

DAY 7

Morning Intention

Take a breath before you begin.

What am I noticing in myself this morning? (Thoughts, emotions, body sensations—anything that stands out.)

_____

_____

_____

Mood
How do you feel right now?
(Circle the one that represents how you feel.)

Energy Level
(Just notice—this isn't about motivation.)

How do I want to feel today?
(Write a word or phrase, or circle one.)

CALM • LIGHTER • STEADY • CONFIDENT
SAFE • FOCUSED • MYSELF

_____

_____

Today's Affirmation or Intention
(Keep it simple. One sentence is enough.)

_____

_____

_____

Today, I give myself permission to take this one step at a time.

Evening Reflection

You made it through the day. That matters.

Mood
How did you feel overall today?

What challenged me today?
(Externally or internally—both count.)

_____

_____

_____

What helped me feel even a little stronger or lighter today? (Small things matter more than you think.)

_____

_____

_____

One thing I'm grateful for today:
(It can be about yourself, someone else, or a quiet moment.)

_____

_____

_____

Gentle Reminder: *If today felt heavy, that doesn't mean you failed. It means you showed up—and that's enough for today.*

TODAY'S LETTING-GO PRACTICE: Notice the Lightness

This is your End-of-Week Reflection. The work of facing pain is difficult. Your act of showing up and acknowledging your truth is a victory. What is one word that describes the strength you've shown this week? What pain did you acknowledge?

_____

_____

_____

_____

_____

_____

_____

_____

YOGA POSE: Supine Twist

Releases spine/lower back tension, promotes relaxation, which can be helpful when confronting difficult emotions.

BREATHWORK EXERCISE: Sighing Breath

Releases stress, promotes immediate relaxation, and can help shift emotional states when facing pain.

See appendix at the back of the book for more details
on Yoga Poses and Breathwork Exercises.

Naming my pain
gives me power.

Naming Toxic Triggers

DAY 8

Morning Intention

Take a breath before you begin.

What am I noticing in myself this morning? (Thoughts, emotions, body sensations—anything that stands out.)

_____

_____

_____

Mood
How do you feel right now?
(Circle the one that represents how you feel.)

Energy Level
(Just notice—
this isn't about
motivation.)

How do I want to feel today?
(Write a word or phrase, or circle one.)

CALM • LIGHTER • STEADY • CONFIDENT
SAFE • FOCUSED • MYSELF

_____

_____

Today's Affirmation or Intention
(Keep it simple. One sentence is enough.)

_____

_____

_____

*Today, I give myself permission
to take this one step at a time.*

Evening Reflection

*You made it through the day.
That matters.*

Mood
How did you feel overall today?

What challenged me today?
(Externally or internally—both count.)

_____

_____

_____

What helped me feel even a little stronger or lighter today? (Small things matter more than you think.)

_____

_____

_____

One thing I'm grateful for today:
(It can be about yourself, someone else, or a quiet moment.)

_____

_____

_____

Gentle Reminder: *If today felt heavy, that doesn't mean you failed. It means you showed up—and that's enough for today.*

TODAY'S LETTING-GO PRACTICE: Identify the Burden

A trigger is a specific situation, person, or thought that activates your pain. List three triggers that you've noticed. Circle the one you want to focus on understanding and disarming this week. This is your burden.

_____

_____

_____

_____

_____

_____

_____

DAY 9

Morning Intention

Take a breath before you begin.

What am I noticing in myself this morning? (Thoughts, emotions, body sensations—anything that stands out.)

_____

_____

_____

Mood
How do you feel right now?
(Circle the one that represents how you feel.)

Energy Level
(Just notice— this isn't about motivation.)

How do I want to feel today?
(Write a word or phrase, or circle one.)

CALM • LIGHTER • STEADY • CONFIDENT
SAFE • FOCUSED • MYSELF

_____

_____

Today's Affirmation or Intention
(Keep it simple. One sentence is enough.)

_____

_____

_____

Today, I give myself permission to take this one step at a time.

Evening Reflection

You made it through the day. That matters.

Mood
How did you feel overall today?

What challenged me today?
(Externally or internally—both count.)

_____

_____

_____

What helped me feel even a little stronger or lighter today? (Small things matter more than you think.)

_____

_____

_____

One thing I'm grateful for today:
(It can be about yourself, someone else, or a quiet moment.)

_____

_____

Gentle Reminder: *If today felt heavy, that doesn't mean you failed. It means you showed up—and that's enough for today.*

TODAY'S LETTING-GO PRACTICE: Write to Understand

Write about the trigger you chose yesterday. When does it usually appear? What specific feelings or memories does it bring to the surface? Explore the "why" behind this trigger without judgment.

_____

_____

_____

_____

_____

_____

_____

DAY 10

Morning Intention

Take a breath before you begin.

What am I noticing in myself this morning? (Thoughts, emotions, body sensations—anything that stands out.)

_____

_____

_____

Mood
How do you feel right now?
(Circle the one that represents how you feel.)

Energy Level
(Just notice—this isn't about motivation.)

How do I want to feel today?
(Write a word or phrase, or circle one.)

CALM • LIGHTER • STEADY • CONFIDENT
SAFE • FOCUSED • MYSELF

_____

_____

Today's Affirmation or Intention
(Keep it simple. One sentence is enough.)

_____

_____

_____

Today, I give myself permission to take this one step at a time.

Evening Reflection

You made it through the day. That matters.

Mood
How did you feel overall today?

What challenged me today?
(Externally or internally—both count.)

_____

_____

_____

What helped me feel even a little stronger or lighter today? (Small things matter more than you think.)

_____

_____

_____

One thing I'm grateful for today:
(It can be about yourself, someone else, or a quiet moment.)

_____

_____

_____

Gentle Reminder: *If today felt heavy, that doesn't mean you failed. It means you showed up—and that's enough for today.*

TODAY'S LETTING-GO PRACTICE: Act of Release

Today's action is a grounding technique. If you encounter your trigger or feel it rising, plant your feet firmly on the floor. Take one slow breath and name three things you can see in the room. This physical act pulls your focus from the internal trigger to the neutral, external world.

DAY 11

Morning Intention

Take a breath before you begin.

What am I noticing in myself this morning? (Thoughts, emotions, body sensations—anything that stands out.)

_____

_____

_____

Mood
How do you feel right now?
(Circle the one that represents how you feel.)

Energy Level
(Just notice—this isn't about motivation.)

How do I want to feel today?
(Write a word or phrase, or circle one.)

CALM • LIGHTER • STEADY • CONFIDENT
SAFE • FOCUSED • MYSELF

_____

_____

Today's Affirmation or Intention
(Keep it simple. One sentence is enough.)

_____

_____

_____

Today, I give myself permission to take this one step at a time.

Evening Reflection

You made it through the day. That matters.

Mood
How did you feel overall today?

What challenged me today?
(Externally or internally—both count.)

_____

_____

_____

What helped me feel even a little stronger or lighter today? (Small things matter more than you think.)

_____

_____

_____

One thing I'm grateful for today:
(It can be about yourself, someone else, or a quiet moment.)

_____

_____

_____

Gentle Reminder: *If today felt heavy, that doesn't mean you failed. It means you showed up—and that's enough for today.*

TODAY'S LETTING-GO PRACTICE: Mindful Detachment

Close your eyes and visualize your trigger as a single word floating in front of you. For one minute, just observe the word. Notice its shape and size. See if you can imagine it gently drifting away, like a balloon into the sky, without getting pulled into the emotion it represents.

DAY 12

Morning Intention

Take a breath before you begin.

What am I noticing in myself this morning? (Thoughts, emotions, body sensations—anything that stands out.)

_____

_____

_____

Mood
How do you feel right now?
(Circle the one that represents how you feel.)

Energy Level
(Just notice—this isn't about motivation.)

How do I want to feel today?
(Write a word or phrase, or circle one.)

CALM • LIGHTER • STEADY • CONFIDENT
SAFE • FOCUSED • MYSELF

_____

_____

Today's Affirmation or Intention
(Keep it simple. One sentence is enough.)

_____

_____

_____

Today, I give myself permission to take this one step at a time.

Evening Reflection

*You made it through the day.
That matters.*

Mood
How did you feel overall today?

What challenged me today?
(Externally or internally—both count.)

_____

_____

_____

What helped me feel even a little stronger or lighter today? (Small things matter more than you think.)

_____

_____

_____

One thing I'm grateful for today:
(It can be about yourself, someone else, or a quiet moment.)

_____

_____

_____

Gentle Reminder: *If today felt heavy, that doesn't mean you failed. It means you showed up—and that's enough for today.*

TODAY'S LETTING-GO PRACTICE:
Reclaim Your Peace (Boundaries)

Revisit your writing from Day 9. Think about when your trigger tends to appear. What is one small way you can create distance from your trigger today? Examples: Mute a word on social media, change the subject in a conversation, or choose a different route on your walk.

_____

_____

_____

_____

_____

_____

_____

DAY 13

Morning Intention

Take a breath before you begin.

What am I noticing in myself this morning? (Thoughts, emotions, body sensations—anything that stands out.)

_____

_____

_____

Mood
How do you feel right now?
(Circle the one that represents how you feel.)

Energy Level
(Just notice—this isn't about motivation.)

How do I want to feel today?
(Write a word or phrase, or circle one.)

CALM • LIGHTER • STEADY • CONFIDENT
SAFE • FOCUSED • MYSELF

_____

_____

Today's Affirmation or Intention
(Keep it simple. One sentence is enough.)

_____

_____

_____

Today, I give myself permission to take this one step at a time.

Evening Reflection

You made it through the day. That matters.

Mood
How did you feel overall today?

What challenged me today?
(Externally or internally—both count.)

_____

_____

_____

What helped me feel even a little stronger or lighter today? (Small things matter more than you think.)

_____

_____

_____

One thing I'm grateful for today:
(It can be about yourself, someone else, or a quiet moment.)

_____

_____

_____

Gentle Reminder: *If today felt heavy, that doesn't mean you failed. It means you showed up—and that's enough for today.*

TODAY'S LETTING-GO PRACTICE: Express and Externalize

Give your trigger a physical form, but not a scary one. If your trigger were a cartoon character, what would it look like? Silly? Annoying? Grumpy? Doodle it on a piece of paper. Giving it a character separates it from you and can reduce its power.

DAY 14

Morning Intention

Take a breath before you begin.

What am I noticing in myself this morning? (Thoughts, emotions, body sensations—anything that stands out.)

_____

_____

_____

Mood
How do you feel right now?
(Circle the one that represents how you feel.)

Energy Level
(Just notice—this isn't about motivation.)

How do I want to feel today?
(Write a word or phrase, or circle one.)

CALM • LIGHTER • STEADY • CONFIDENT
SAFE • FOCUSED • MYSELF

_____

_____

Today's Affirmation or Intention
(Keep it simple. One sentence is enough.)

_____

_____

_____

Today, I give myself permission to take this one step at a time.

Evening Reflection

You made it through the day. That matters.

Mood
How did you feel overall today?

What challenged me today?
(Externally or internally—both count.)

_____

_____

_____

What helped me feel even a little stronger or lighter today? (Small things matter more than you think.)

_____

_____

_____

One thing I'm grateful for today:
(It can be about yourself, someone else, or a quiet moment.)

_____

_____

_____

Gentle Reminder: *If today felt heavy, that doesn't mean you failed. It means you showed up—and that's enough for today.*

TODAY'S LETTING-GO PRACTICE: Notice the Lightness

This is your End-of-Week Reflection. The mantra states: "Naming my pain gives me power." How did it feel to name and observe your trigger this week? Which trigger had the most control over you, and do you feel you've gained any power back by focusing on it?

_____

_____

_____

_____

_____

_____

_____

_____

YOGA POSE: Easy Pose

Promotes calmness/mental clarity, ideal for meditation/breathwork, which can help in observing and understanding triggers without judgment.

BREATHWORK EXERCISE: The 5-4-3-2-1 Technique

Grounding exercise that reduces anxiety and brings focus, useful for interrupting overwhelming thoughts caused by triggers.

See appendix at the back of the book for more details
on Yoga Poses and Breathwork Exercises.

My voice deserves
to be heard.

Speaking the Truth

DAY 15

Morning Intention

Take a breath before you begin.

What am I noticing in myself this morning? (Thoughts, emotions, body sensations—anything that stands out.)

_____

_____

_____

Mood
How do you feel right now?
(Circle the one that represents how you feel.)

Energy Level
(Just notice—this isn't about motivation.)

How do I want to feel today?
(Write a word or phrase, or circle one.)

CALM • LIGHTER • STEADY • CONFIDENT
SAFE • FOCUSED • MYSELF

_____

_____

Today's Affirmation or Intention
(Keep it simple. One sentence is enough.)

_____

_____

_____

Today, I give myself permission to take this one step at a time.

Evening Reflection

You made it through the day. That matters.

Mood
How did you feel overall today?

What challenged me today?
(Externally or internally—both count.)

_____

_____

_____

What helped me feel even a little stronger or lighter today? (Small things matter more than you think.)

_____

_____

_____

One thing I'm grateful for today:
(It can be about yourself, someone else, or a quiet moment.)

_____

_____

_____

Gentle Reminder: *If today felt heavy, that doesn't mean you failed. It means you showed up—and that's enough for today.*

TODAY'S LETTING-GO PRACTICE: Identify the Burden

The burden this week is silence. What is one truth you have been holding in, afraid or unwilling to speak? Identify the unspoken words that feel heavy. This is your focus for the week.

_____

_____

_____

_____

_____

_____

_____

DAY 16

Morning Intention

Take a breath before you begin.

What am I noticing in myself this morning? (Thoughts, emotions, body sensations—anything that stands out.)

_____

_____

_____

Mood
How do you feel right now?
(Circle the one that represents how you feel.)

Energy Level
(Just notice—this isn't about motivation.)

How do I want to feel today?
(Write a word or phrase, or circle one.)

CALM • LIGHTER • STEADY • CONFIDENT
SAFE • FOCUSED • MYSELF

_____

_____

Today's Affirmation or Intention
(Keep it simple. One sentence is enough.)

_____

_____

_____

Today, I give myself permission to take this one step at a time.

Evening Reflection

*You made it through the day.
That matters.*

Mood
How did you feel overall today?

What challenged me today?
(Externally or internally—both count.)

_____

_____

_____

What helped me feel even a little stronger or lighter today? (Small things matter more than you think.)

_____

_____

_____

One thing I'm grateful for today:
(It can be about yourself, someone else, or a quiet moment.)

_____

_____

_____

Gentle Reminder: *If today felt heavy, that doesn't mean you failed. It means you showed up—and that's enough for today.*

TODAY'S LETTING-GO PRACTICE: Write to Understand

Today you will write a truth letter. Write a letter to a person
(or to yourself) expressing the truth you identified yesterday.
This letter is for you and will not be sent. Allow yourself to be
completely honest.

_____

_____

_____

_____

_____

_____

_____

_____

DAY 17

Morning Intention

Take a breath before you begin.

What am I noticing in myself this morning? (Thoughts, emotions, body sensations—anything that stands out.)

_____

_____

_____

Mood
How do you feel right now?
(Circle the one that represents how you feel.)

Energy Level
(Just notice—this isn't about motivation.)

How do I want to feel today?
(Write a word or phrase, or circle one.)

CALM • LIGHTER • STEADY • CONFIDENT
SAFE • FOCUSED • MYSELF

_____

_____

Today's Affirmation or Intention
(Keep it simple. One sentence is enough.)

_____

_____

_____

Today, I give myself permission to take this one step at a time.

Evening Reflection

*You made it through the day.
That matters.*

Mood
How did you feel overall today?

What challenged me today?
(Externally or internally—both count.)

_____

_____

_____

What helped me feel even a little stronger or lighter today? (Small things matter more than you think.)

_____

_____

_____

One thing I'm grateful for today:
(It can be about yourself, someone else, or a quiet moment.)

_____

_____

_____

Gentle Reminder: *If today felt heavy, that doesn't mean you failed. It means you showed up—and that's enough for today.*

TODAY'S LETTING-GO PRACTICE: Act of Release

Give your truth a voice. Read one single sentence from yesterday's truth letter out loud to an empty room. Feel the physical vibration of your voice speaking the words. Notice how it feels to have the truth exist in the air, not just in your head.

DAY 18

Morning Intention

Take a breath before you begin.

What am I noticing in myself this morning? (Thoughts, emotions, body sensations—anything that stands out.)

_____

_____

_____

Mood
How do you feel right now?
(Circle the one that represents how you feel.)

Energy Level
(Just notice—
this isn't about
motivation.)

How do I want to feel today?
(Write a word or phrase, or circle one.)

CALM • LIGHTER • STEADY • CONFIDENT
SAFE • FOCUSED • MYSELF

_____

_____

Today's Affirmation or Intention
(Keep it simple. One sentence is enough.)

_____

_____

_____

*Today, I give myself permission
to take this one step at a time.*

Evening Reflection

*You made it through the day.
That matters.*

Mood
How did you feel overall today?

What challenged me today?
(Externally or internally—both count.)

_____

_____

_____

What helped me feel even a little stronger or lighter today? (Small things matter more than you think.)

_____

_____

_____

One thing I'm grateful for today:
(It can be about yourself, someone else, or a quiet moment.)

_____

_____

_____

Gentle Reminder: *If today felt heavy, that doesn't mean you failed. It means you showed up—and that's enough for today.*

TODAY'S LETTING-GO PRACTICE: Mindful Detachment

After speaking a truth, even to yourself, feelings of fear or
vulnerability can arise. Take a moment to scan your body. Where
do you feel this vulnerability? In your stomach? Your chest? Your
throat? Simply notice the physical sensation without labeling it
"bad." Observe it with gentle curiosity.

_____

_____

_____

_____

_____

_____

_____

DAY 19

Morning Intention

Take a breath before you begin.

What am I noticing in myself this morning? (Thoughts, emotions, body sensations—anything that stands out.)

_____

_____

_____

Mood
How do you feel right now?
(Circle the one that represents how you feel.)

Energy Level
(Just notice— this isn't about motivation.)

How do I want to feel today?
(Write a word or phrase, or circle one.)

CALM • LIGHTER • STEADY • CONFIDENT
SAFE • FOCUSED • MYSELF

_____

_____

Today's Affirmation or Intention
(Keep it simple. One sentence is enough.)

_____

_____

_____

Today, I give myself permission to take this one step at a time.

Evening Reflection

You made it through the day. That matters.

Mood
How did you feel overall today?

What challenged me today?
(Externally or internally—both count.)

_____

_____

_____

What helped me feel even a little stronger or lighter today? (Small things matter more than you think.)

_____

_____

_____

One thing I'm grateful for today:
(It can be about yourself, someone else, or a quiet moment.)

_____

_____

_____

Gentle Reminder: *If today felt heavy, that doesn't mean you failed. It means you showed up—and that's enough for today.*

TODAY'S LETTING-GO PRACTICE:
Reclaim Your Peace (Boundaries)

Speaking your truth also means knowing when not to speak. A boundary can be choosing not to share your feelings with someone who is unsafe or unreceptive. Today, practice the boundary of "no explanation needed." Release the need to justify your feelings to others.

DAY 20

Morning Intention

Take a breath before you begin.

What am I noticing in myself this morning? (Thoughts, emotions, body sensations—anything that stands out.)

_____

_____

_____

Mood
How do you feel right now?
(Circle the one that represents how you feel.)

Energy Level
(Just notice—this isn't about motivation.)

How do I want to feel today?
(Write a word or phrase, or circle one.)

CALM • LIGHTER • STEADY • CONFIDENT
SAFE • FOCUSED • MYSELF

_____

_____

Today's Affirmation or Intention
(Keep it simple. One sentence is enough.)

_____

_____

_____

Today, I give myself permission to take this one step at a time.

Evening Reflection

*You made it through the day.
That matters.*

Mood
How did you feel overall today?

What challenged me today?
(Externally or internally—both count.)

_____

_____

_____

What helped me feel even a little stronger or lighter today? (Small things matter more than you think.)

_____

_____

_____

One thing I'm grateful for today:
(It can be about yourself, someone else, or a quiet moment.)

_____

_____

_____

Gentle Reminder: *If today felt heavy, that doesn't mean you failed. It means you showed up—and that's enough for today.*

TODAY'S LETTING-GO PRACTICE: Express and Externalize

Find a song where an artist speaks their truth with power and
passion. Listen to it carefully. Which lyric stands out to you
the most? Write it down. Let someone else's courage amplify
your own.

_____

_____

_____

_____

_____

_____

_____

DAY 21

Morning Intention

Take a breath before you begin.

What am I noticing in myself this morning? (Thoughts, emotions, body sensations—anything that stands out.)

_____

_____

_____

Mood
How do you feel right now?
(Circle the one that represents how you feel.)

Energy Level
(Just notice—this isn't about motivation.)

How do I want to feel today?
(Write a word or phrase, or circle one.)

CALM • LIGHTER • STEADY • CONFIDENT
SAFE • FOCUSED • MYSELF

_____

_____

Today's Affirmation or Intention
(Keep it simple. One sentence is enough.)

_____

_____

_____

Today, I give myself permission to take this one step at a time.

Evening Reflection

You made it through the day. That matters.

Mood
How did you feel overall today?

What challenged me today?
(Externally or internally—both count.)

_____

_____

_____

What helped me feel even a little stronger or lighter today? (Small things matter more than you think.)

_____

_____

_____

One thing I'm grateful for today:
(It can be about yourself, someone else, or a quiet moment.)

_____

_____

_____

Gentle Reminder: *If today felt heavy, that doesn't mean you failed. It means you showed up—and that's enough for today.*

TODAY'S LETTING-GO PRACTICE: Notice the Lightness

This is your End-of-Week Reflection. How did it feel to express your truth this week, even if only to yourself? Did the act of writing and speaking the words lessen their weight? Acknowledge the courage it took to honor your voice.

_____

_____

_____

_____

_____

_____

_____

YOGA POSE: Cat-Cow Pose

Warms spine, improves flexibility, links breath/movement, which can help in finding physical and emotional fluidity to express oneself.

BREATHWORK EXERCISE: Lion's Breath

Releases jaw/face tension, energizes, and relieves frustration/stress, which can be beneficial when preparing to speak one's truth.

See appendix at the back of the book for more details
on Yoga Poses and Breathwork Exercises.

I forgive myself for being human.

Releasing Guilt

DAY 22

Morning Intention

Take a breath before you begin.

What am I noticing in myself this morning? (Thoughts, emotions, body sensations—anything that stands out.)

_____

_____

_____

Mood
How do you feel right now?
(Circle the one that represents how you feel.)

Energy Level
(Just notice—
this isn't about
motivation.)

How do I want to feel today?
(Write a word or phrase, or circle one.)

CALM • LIGHTER • STEADY • CONFIDENT
SAFE • FOCUSED • MYSELF

_____

_____

Today's Affirmation or Intention
(Keep it simple. One sentence is enough.)

_____

_____

_____

*Today, I give myself permission
to take this one step at a time.*

Evening Reflection

*You made it through the day.
That matters.*

Mood
How did you feel overall today?

What challenged me today?
(Externally or internally—both count.)

_____

_____

_____

What helped me feel even a little stronger or lighter today? (Small things matter more than you think.)

_____

_____

_____

One thing I'm grateful for today:
(It can be about yourself, someone else, or a quiet moment.)

_____

_____

_____

Gentle Reminder: *If today felt heavy, that doesn't mean you failed. It means you showed up—and that's enough for today.*

TODAY'S LETTING-GO PRACTICE: Identify the Burden

Guilt often lives in thoughts of "I should have . . ." or "I shouldn't have . . ." Identify one specific guilty thought that is weighing on you. This is the burden you will focus on releasing this week.

_____

_____

_____

_____

_____

_____

_____

DAY 23

Morning Intention

Take a breath before you begin.

What am I noticing in myself this morning? (Thoughts, emotions, body sensations—anything that stands out.)

_____

_____

_____

Mood
How do you feel right now?
(Circle the one that represents how you feel.)

Energy Level
(Just notice—this isn't about motivation.)

How do I want to feel today?
(Write a word or phrase, or circle one.)

CALM • LIGHTER • STEADY • CONFIDENT
SAFE • FOCUSED • MYSELF

_____

_____

Today's Affirmation or Intention
(Keep it simple. One sentence is enough.)

_____

_____

_____

Today, I give myself permission to take this one step at a time.

Evening Reflection

You made it through the day. That matters.

Mood
How did you feel overall today?

What challenged me today?
(Externally or internally—both count.)

_____

_____

_____

What helped me feel even a little stronger or lighter today? (Small things matter more than you think.)

_____

_____

_____

One thing I'm grateful for today:
(It can be about yourself, someone else, or a quiet moment.)

_____

_____

_____

Gentle Reminder: *If today felt heavy, that doesn't mean you failed. It means you showed up—and that's enough for today.*

TODAY'S LETTING-GO PRACTICE: Write to Understand

Write about the guilty feeling you identified yesterday. Where did it come from? What expectations—from yourself or others— are attached to it? What do you believe holding onto this guilt is accomplishing?

_____

_____

_____

_____

_____

_____

_____

_____

DAY 24

Morning Intention

Take a breath before you begin.

What am I noticing in myself this morning? (Thoughts, emotions, body sensations—anything that stands out.)

_____

_____

_____

Mood
How do you feel right now?
(Circle the one that represents how you feel.)

Energy Level
(Just notice—
this isn't about
motivation.)

How do I want to feel today?
(Write a word or phrase, or circle one.)

CALM • LIGHTER • STEADY • CONFIDENT
SAFE • FOCUSED • MYSELF

_____

_____

Today's Affirmation or Intention
(Keep it simple. One sentence is enough.)

_____

_____

_____

*Today, I give myself permission
to take this one step at a time.*

Evening Reflection

*You made it through the day.
That matters.*

Mood
How did you feel overall today?

What challenged me today?
(Externally or internally—both count.)

_____

_____

_____

What helped me feel even a little stronger or lighter today? (Small things matter more than you think.)

_____

_____

_____

One thing I'm grateful for today:
(It can be about yourself, someone else, or a quiet moment.)

_____

_____

_____

Gentle Reminder: *If today felt heavy, that doesn't mean you failed. It means you showed up—and that's enough for today.*

TODAY'S LETTING-GO PRACTICE: Act of Release

Today you will perform a release ritual. Write your guilty thought(s) or burden on a piece of paper. When you are ready, safely destroy it by ripping it up or burning it. As you do, imagine the weight of that guilt being released.

_____

_____

_____

_____

_____

_____

_____

_____

DAY 25

Morning Intention

Take a breath before you begin.

What am I noticing in myself this morning? (Thoughts, emotions, body sensations—anything that stands out.)

_____

_____

_____

Mood
How do you feel right now?
(Circle the one that represents how you feel.)

Energy Level
(Just notice— this isn't about motivation.)

How do I want to feel today?
(Write a word or phrase, or circle one.)

CALM • LIGHTER • STEADY • CONFIDENT
SAFE • FOCUSED • MYSELF

_____

_____

Today's Affirmation or Intention
(Keep it simple. One sentence is enough.)

_____

_____

_____

*Today, I give myself permission
to take this one step at a time.*

Evening Reflection

*You made it through the day.
That matters.*

Mood
How did you feel overall today?

What challenged me today?
(Externally or internally—both count.)

_____

_____

_____

What helped me feel even a little stronger or lighter today? (Small things matter more than you think.)

_____

_____

_____

One thing I'm grateful for today:
(It can be about yourself, someone else, or a quiet moment.)

_____

_____

_____

Gentle Reminder: *If today felt heavy, that doesn't mean you failed. It means you showed up—and that's enough for today.*

TODAY'S LETTING-GO PRACTICE: Mindful Detachment

When the guilty thought returns, as it might, practice noticing it without getting caught in it. Silently label the thought as "guilt" or simply "thinking." Acknowledge its presence and then gently guide your attention back to your breath.

DAY 26

Morning Intention

Take a breath before you begin.

What am I noticing in myself this morning? (Thoughts, emotions, body sensations—anything that stands out.)

_____

_____

_____

Mood
How do you feel right now?
(Circle the one that represents how you feel.)

Energy Level
(Just notice— this isn't about motivation.)

How do I want to feel today?
(Write a word or phrase, or circle one.)

CALM • LIGHTER • STEADY • CONFIDENT
SAFE • FOCUSED • MYSELF

_____

_____

Today's Affirmation or Intention
(Keep it simple. One sentence is enough.)

_____

_____

_____

Today, I give myself permission to take this one step at a time.

Evening Reflection

You made it through the day. That matters.

Mood
How did you feel overall today?

What challenged me today?
(Externally or internally—both count.)

_____

_____

_____

What helped me feel even a little stronger or lighter today? (Small things matter more than you think.)

_____

_____

_____

One thing I'm grateful for today:
(It can be about yourself, someone else, or a quiet moment.)

_____

_____

_____

Gentle Reminder: *If today felt heavy, that doesn't mean you failed. It means you showed up—and that's enough for today.*

TODAY'S LETTING-GO PRACTICE:
Reclaim Your Peace (Boundaries)

Set a boundary against self-punishment. If you find yourself replaying the guilty thought, gently interrupt the loop. Say to yourself, "I am allowed to move on." Then, shift your focus to something in the present moment for one minute (e.g., the feeling of your feet on the floor).

DAY 27

Morning Intention

Take a breath before you begin.

What am I noticing in myself this morning? (Thoughts, emotions, body sensations—anything that stands out.)

_____

_____

_____

Mood
How do you feel right now?
(Circle the one that represents how you feel.)

Energy Level
(Just notice—
this isn't about
motivation.)

How do I want to feel today?
(Write a word or phrase, or circle one.)

CALM • LIGHTER • STEADY • CONFIDENT
SAFE • FOCUSED • MYSELF

_____

_____

Today's Affirmation or Intention
(Keep it simple. One sentence is enough.)

_____

_____

_____

*Today, I give myself permission
to take this one step at a time.*

Evening Reflection

*You made it through the day.
That matters.*

Mood
How did you feel overall today?

What challenged me today?
(Externally or internally—both count.)

_____

_____

_____

What helped me feel even a little stronger or lighter today? (Small things matter more than you think.)

_____

_____

_____

One thing I'm grateful for today:
(It can be about yourself, someone else, or a quiet moment.)

_____

_____

_____

Gentle Reminder: *If today felt heavy, that doesn't mean you failed. It means you showed up—and that's enough for today.*

TODAY'S LETTING-GO PRACTICE: Express and Externalize

Think of a time you genuinely forgave someone else. What did that feeling of compassion look like or feel like? Choose a color that represents it. Spend a few minutes doodling with that color, filling a space on your page with the color of forgiveness.

_____

_____

_____

_____

_____

_____

_____

DAY 28

Morning Intention	Evening Reflection

Take a breath before you begin.

You made it through the day. That matters.

What am I noticing in myself this morning? (Thoughts, emotions, body sensations—anything that stands out.)

_____

_____

_____

Mood
How did you feel overall today?

What challenged me today?
(Externally or internally—both count.)

_____

_____

_____

Mood
How do you feel right now?
(Circle the one that represents how you feel.)

What helped me feel even a little stronger or lighter today? (Small things matter more than you think.)

_____

_____

_____

Energy Level
(Just notice—
this isn't about
motivation.)

How do I want to feel today?
(Write a word or phrase, or circle one.)

CALM • LIGHTER • STEADY • CONFIDENT
SAFE • FOCUSED • MYSELF

_____

_____

One thing I'm grateful for today:
(It can be about yourself, someone else, or a quiet moment.)

_____

_____

_____

Today's Affirmation or Intention
(Keep it simple. One sentence is enough.)

_____

_____

_____

Today, I give myself permission to take this one step at a time.

Gentle Reminder: *If today felt heavy, that doesn't mean you failed. It means you showed up—and that's enough for today.*

TODAY'S LETTING-GO PRACTICE: Notice the Lightness

This is your End-of-Week Reflection. Reflect on this week's mantra: "I forgive myself for being human." How did the release ritual on Day 24 feel? What guilt did you let go of, even just a little?

_____

_____

_____

_____

_____

_____

_____

YOGA POSE: Reclining Butterfly

Gently opens hips/groin, calms mind, relieves stress/mild depression, offering a gentle release for feelings of guilt.

BREATHWORK EXERCISE: Resonant Breathing

Balances nervous system, promotes relaxation, and reduces stress, aiding in the gentle process of self-forgiveness and releasing guilt.

See appendix at the back of the book for more details on Yoga Poses and Breathwork Exercises.

REFLECTION ON THE PAST 4 WEEKS

What was your biggest insight or breakthrough during the last four weeks?

_____

_____

_____

_____

_____

_____

_____

What challenge did you face, and how did you overcome it (or what did you learn from it)?

_____

_____

_____

_____

_____

_____

_____

REFLECTION ON THE PAST 4 WEEKS

What is one thing you are grateful for from these past four weeks?

_____

_____

_____

_____

_____

_____

_____

How has your sense of peace or understanding of "letting go" evolved?

_____

_____

_____

_____

_____

_____

_____

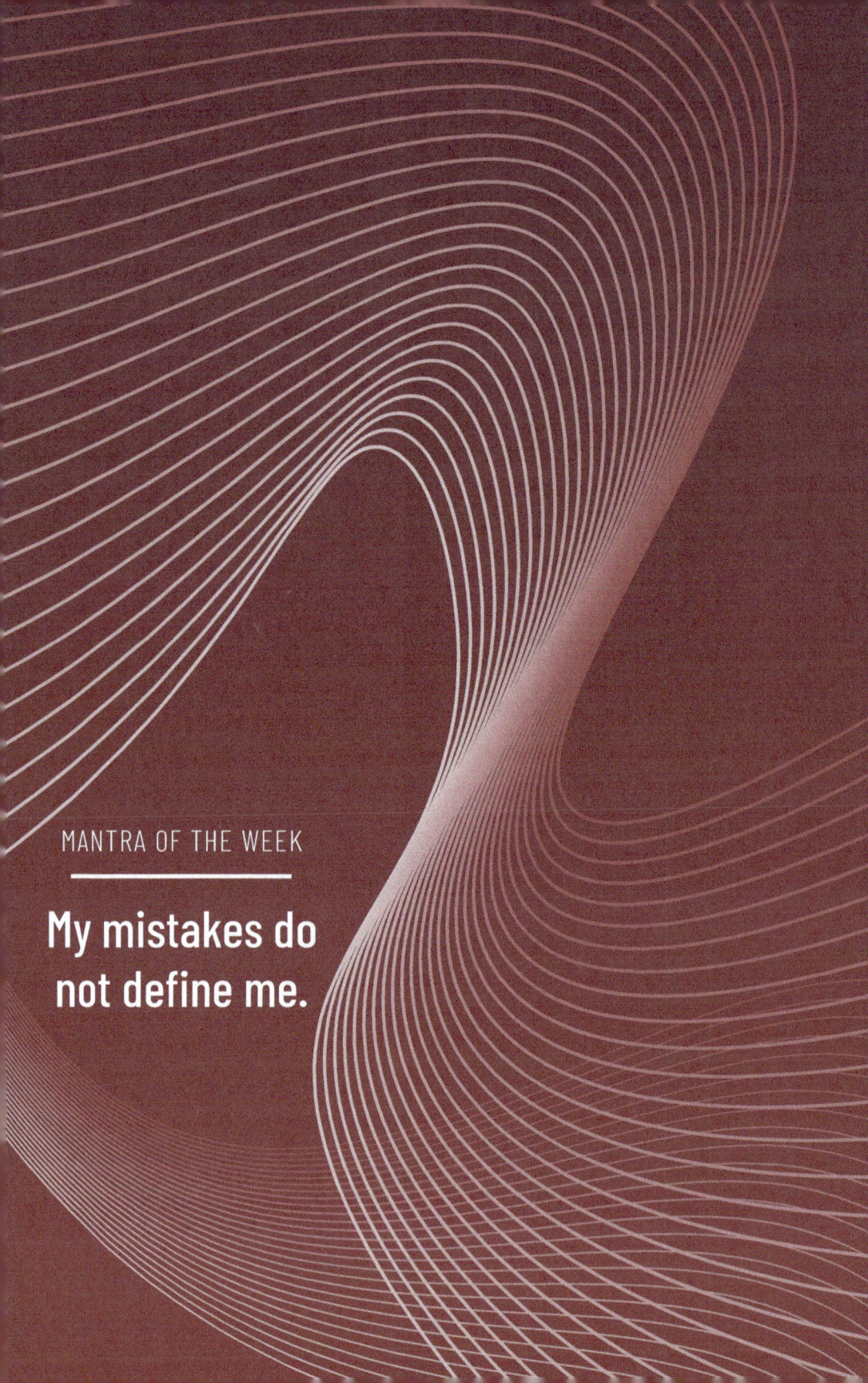

MANTRA OF THE WEEK

My mistakes do
not define me.

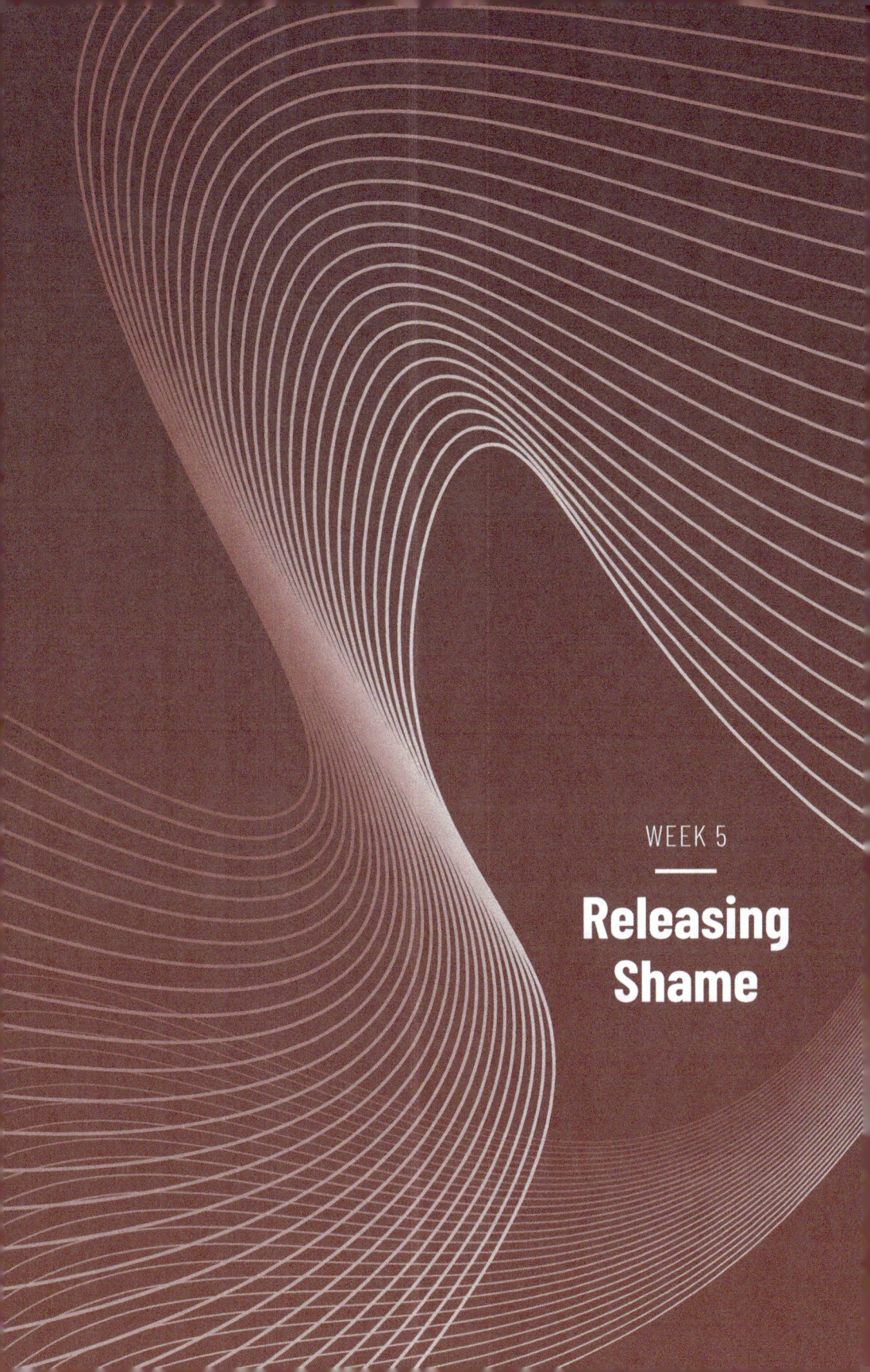

Releasing Shame

DAY 29

Morning Intention

Take a breath before you begin.

What am I noticing in myself this morning? (Thoughts, emotions, body sensations—anything that stands out.)

_____

_____

_____

Mood
How do you feel right now?
(Circle the one that represents how you feel.)

Energy Level
(Just notice—this isn't about motivation.)

How do I want to feel today?
(Write a word or phrase, or circle one.)

CALM • LIGHTER • STEADY • CONFIDENT
SAFE • FOCUSED • MYSELF

_____

_____

Today's Affirmation or Intention
(Keep it simple. One sentence is enough.)

_____

_____

_____

Today, I give myself permission to take this one step at a time.

Evening Reflection

*You made it through the day.
That matters.*

Mood
How did you feel overall today?

What challenged me today?
(Externally or internally—both count.)

_____

_____

_____

What helped me feel even a little stronger or lighter today? (Small things matter more than you think.)

_____

_____

_____

One thing I'm grateful for today:
(It can be about yourself, someone else, or a quiet moment.)

_____

_____

_____

Gentle Reminder: *If today felt heavy, that doesn't mean you failed. It means you showed up—and that's enough for today.*

TODAY'S LETTING-GO PRACTICE: Identify the Burden

Shame often makes us feel broken or fundamentally flawed. The burden this week is a specific mistake you've made that you keep punishing yourself for. Identify one past action that you are ready to stop letting define you.

_____

_____

_____

_____

_____

_____

_____

DAY 30

Morning Intention

Take a breath before you begin.

What am I noticing in myself this morning? (Thoughts, emotions, body sensations—anything that stands out.)

_____

_____

_____

Mood
How do you feel right now?
(Circle the one that represents how you feel.)

Energy Level
(Just notice— this isn't about motivation.)

How do I want to feel today?
(Write a word or phrase, or circle one.)

CALM • LIGHTER • STEADY • CONFIDENT
SAFE • FOCUSED • MYSELF

_____

_____

Today's Affirmation or Intention
(Keep it simple. One sentence is enough.)

_____

_____

_____

Today, I give myself permission to take this one step at a time.

Evening Reflection

You made it through the day. That matters.

Mood
How did you feel overall today?

What challenged me today?
(Externally or internally—both count.)

_____

_____

_____

What helped me feel even a little stronger or lighter today? (Small things matter more than you think.)

_____

_____

_____

One thing I'm grateful for today:
(It can be about yourself, someone else, or a quiet moment.)

_____

_____

_____

Gentle Reminder: *If today felt heavy, that doesn't mean you failed. It means you showed up—and that's enough for today.*

TODAY'S LETTING-GO PRACTICE: Write to Understand

Write the story of the mistake you identified yesterday, but as an observer, not a judge. Describe the event. Then, write about what you learned from it. The goal is to separate the action (what you did) from your identity (who you are).

_____

_____

_____

_____

_____

_____

_____

_____

DAY 31

Morning Intention

Take a breath before you begin.

What am I noticing in myself this morning? (Thoughts, emotions, body sensations—anything that stands out.)

_____

_____

_____

Mood
How do you feel right now?
(Circle the one that represents how you feel.)

Energy Level
(Just notice—
this isn't about
motivation.)

How do I want to feel today?
(Write a word or phrase, or circle one.)

CALM • LIGHTER • STEADY • CONFIDENT
SAFE • FOCUSED • MYSELF

_____

_____

Today's Affirmation or Intention
(Keep it simple. One sentence is enough.)

_____

_____

_____

*Today, I give myself permission
to take this one step at a time.*

Evening Reflection

*You made it through the day.
That matters.*

Mood
How did you feel overall today?

What challenged me today?
(Externally or internally—both count.)

_____

_____

_____

What helped me feel even a little stronger or lighter today? (Small things matter more than you think.)

_____

_____

_____

One thing I'm grateful for today:
(It can be about yourself, someone else, or a quiet moment.)

_____

_____

_____

Gentle Reminder: *If today felt heavy, that doesn't mean you failed. It means you showed up—and that's enough for today.*

TODAY'S LETTING-GO PRACTICE: Act of Release

Today you will do a stone release. Find a small stone. Hold it and imagine transferring the heavy feeling of shame into it. When you're ready, throw the stone into a body of water, or simply leave it on the ground and walk away, physically separating yourself from the burden.

DAY 32

Morning Intention

Take a breath before you begin.

What am I noticing in myself this morning? (Thoughts, emotions, body sensations—anything that stands out.)

_____

_____

_____

Mood
How do you feel right now?
(Circle the one that represents how you feel.)

Energy Level
(Just notice—
this isn't about
motivation.)

How do I want to feel today?
(Write a word or phrase, or circle one.)

CALM • LIGHTER • STEADY • CONFIDENT
SAFE • FOCUSED • MYSELF

_____

_____

Today's Affirmation or Intention
(Keep it simple. One sentence is enough.)

_____

_____

_____

*Today, I give myself permission
to take this one step at a time.*

Evening Reflection

*You made it through the day.
That matters.*

Mood
How did you feel overall today?

What challenged me today?
(Externally or internally—both count.)

_____

_____

_____

What helped me feel even a little stronger or lighter today? (Small things matter more than you think.)

_____

_____

_____

One thing I'm grateful for today:
(It can be about yourself, someone else, or a quiet moment.)

_____

_____

_____

Gentle Reminder: *If today felt heavy, that doesn't mean you failed. It means you showed up—and that's enough for today.*

TODAY'S LETTING-GO PRACTICE: Mindful Detachment

Shame can feel like a hot, physical sensation. When you feel a wave of shame today, try to notice where it shows up in your body (e.g., a flushed face, a sinking feeling in your stomach). Name the physical sensation without judgment. This creates distance from the shaming story in your mind.

_____

_____

_____

_____

_____

_____

_____

DAY 33

Morning Intention

Take a breath before you begin.

What am I noticing in myself this morning? (Thoughts, emotions, body sensations—anything that stands out.)

_____

_____

_____

Mood
How do you feel right now?
(Circle the one that represents how you feel.)

Energy Level
(Just notice—this isn't about motivation.)

How do I want to feel today?
(Write a word or phrase, or circle one.)

CALM • LIGHTER • STEADY • CONFIDENT
SAFE • FOCUSED • MYSELF

_____

_____

Today's Affirmation or Intention
(Keep it simple. One sentence is enough.)

_____

_____

Today, I give myself permission to take this one step at a time.

Evening Reflection

You made it through the day. That matters.

Mood
How did you feel overall today?

What challenged me today?
(Externally or internally—both count.)

_____

_____

_____

What helped me feel even a little stronger or lighter today? (Small things matter more than you think.)

_____

_____

_____

One thing I'm grateful for today:
(It can be about yourself, someone else, or a quiet moment.)

_____

_____

Gentle Reminder: *If today felt heavy, that doesn't mean you failed. It means you showed up—and that's enough for today.*

TODAY'S LETTING-GO PRACTICE:
Reclaim Your Peace (Boundaries)

Set a boundary against the toxic thought "I'm broken." Each time you catch yourself thinking about it, gently but firmly correct it with the phrase, "I am healing." This is a boundary for your own self-talk.

DAY 34

Morning Intention

Take a breath before you begin.

What am I noticing in myself this morning? (Thoughts, emotions, body sensations—anything that stands out.)

_____

_____

_____

Mood
How do you feel right now?
(Circle the one that represents how you feel.)

Energy Level
(Just notice—
this isn't about
motivation.)

How do I want to feel today?
(Write a word or phrase, or circle one.)

CALM • LIGHTER • STEADY • CONFIDENT
SAFE • FOCUSED • MYSELF

_____

_____

Today's Affirmation or Intention
(Keep it simple. One sentence is enough.)

_____

_____

_____

*Today, I give myself permission
to take this one step at a time.*

Evening Reflection

*You made it through the day.
That matters.*

Mood
How did you feel overall today?

What challenged me today?
(Externally or internally—both count.)

_____

_____

_____

What helped me feel even a little stronger or lighter today? (Small things matter more than you think.)

_____

_____

_____

One thing I'm grateful for today:
(It can be about yourself, someone else, or a quiet moment.)

_____

_____

_____

Gentle Reminder: *If today felt heavy, that doesn't mean you failed. It means you showed up—and that's enough for today.*

TODAY'S LETTING-GO PRACTICE: Express and Externalize

Shame thrives in secrecy; its opposite is authenticity. Think of one safe person in your life. Imagine telling them one small, true thing about yourself. Write down what you would say. You don't have to send it; the goal is to practice expressing your authentic self.

_____

_____

_____

_____

_____

_____

_____

_____

DAY 35

Morning Intention

Take a breath before you begin.

What am I noticing in myself this morning? (Thoughts, emotions, body sensations—anything that stands out.)

_____

_____

_____

Mood
How do you feel right now?
(Circle the one that represents how you feel.)

Energy Level
(Just notice—this isn't about motivation.)

How do I want to feel today?
(Write a word or phrase, or circle one.)

CALM • LIGHTER • STEADY • CONFIDENT
SAFE • FOCUSED • MYSELF

_____

_____

Today's Affirmation or Intention
(Keep it simple. One sentence is enough.)

_____

_____

_____

Today, I give myself permission to take this one step at a time.

Evening Reflection

*You made it through the day.
That matters.*

Mood
How did you feel overall today?

What challenged me today?
(Externally or internally—both count.)

_____

_____

_____

What helped me feel even a little stronger or lighter today? (Small things matter more than you think.)

_____

_____

_____

One thing I'm grateful for today:
(It can be about yourself, someone else, or a quiet moment.)

_____

_____

_____

Gentle Reminder: *If today felt heavy, that doesn't mean you failed. It means you showed up—and that's enough for today.*

TODAY'S LETTING-GO PRACTICE: Notice the Lightness

This is your End-of-Week Reflection. Reflect on this week's mantra: "My mistakes do not define me." What shame lost power over you this week? How did it feel to acknowledge that you are a human who is healing, not a person who is broken?

_____

_____

_____

_____

_____

_____

_____

_____

YOGA POSE: Standing Forward Bend

Stretches hamstrings/calves/hips, calms brain, relieves stress/mild depression, providing a physical release for the weight of shame.

BREATHWORK EXERCISE: Box Breathing

Calms nerves, reduces stress, improves focus/clarity, which can help in detaching from shaming thoughts and fostering a sense of control.

See appendix at the back of the book for more details
on Yoga Poses and Breathwork Exercises.

I deserve my own compassion.

Self-Forgiveness

DAY 36

Morning Intention

Take a breath before you begin.

What am I noticing in myself this morning? (Thoughts, emotions, body sensations—anything that stands out.)

_____

_____

_____

Mood
How do you feel right now?
(Circle the one that represents how you feel.)

Energy Level
(Just notice—this isn't about motivation.)

How do I want to feel today?
(Write a word or phrase, or circle one.)

CALM • LIGHTER • STEADY • CONFIDENT
SAFE • FOCUSED • MYSELF

_____

_____

Today's Affirmation or Intention
(Keep it simple. One sentence is enough.)

_____

_____

_____

Today, I give myself permission to take this one step at a time.

Evening Reflection

You made it through the day. That matters.

Mood
How did you feel overall today?

What challenged me today?
(Externally or internally—both count.)

_____

_____

_____

What helped me feel even a little stronger or lighter today? (Small things matter more than you think.)

_____

_____

_____

One thing I'm grateful for today:
(It can be about yourself, someone else, or a quiet moment.)

_____

_____

_____

Gentle Reminder: *If today felt heavy, that doesn't mean you failed. It means you showed up—and that's enough for today.*

TODAY'S LETTING-GO PRACTICE: Identify the Burden

The burden this week is a specific judgment you hold against yourself. What is one thing you are finding it hard to forgive yourself for? Name it without judgment.

_____

_____

_____

_____

_____

_____

_____

DAY 37

Morning Intention

Take a breath before you begin.

What am I noticing in myself this morning? (Thoughts, emotions, body sensations—anything that stands out.)

_____

_____

_____

Mood
How do you feel right now?
(Circle the one that represents how you feel.)

Energy Level
(Just notice— this isn't about motivation.)

How do I want to feel today?
(Write a word or phrase, or circle one.)

CALM • LIGHTER • STEADY • CONFIDENT
SAFE • FOCUSED • MYSELF

_____

_____

Today's Affirmation or Intention
(Keep it simple. One sentence is enough.)

_____

_____

_____

Today, I give myself permission to take this one step at a time.

Evening Reflection

You made it through the day. That matters.

Mood
How did you feel overall today?

What challenged me today?
(Externally or internally—both count.)

_____

_____

_____

What helped me feel even a little stronger or lighter today? (Small things matter more than you think.)

_____

_____

_____

One thing I'm grateful for today:
(It can be about yourself, someone else, or a quiet moment.)

_____

_____

_____

Gentle Reminder: *If today felt heavy, that doesn't mean you failed. It means you showed up—and that's enough for today.*

TODAY'S LETTING-GO PRACTICE: Write to Understand

Write about the situation you identified yesterday, but imagine you are writing to a dear friend who went through the same thing. What words of compassion, understanding, and forgiveness would you offer them?

_____

_____

_____

_____

_____

_____

_____

DAY 38

Morning Intention

Take a breath before you begin.

What am I noticing in myself this morning? (Thoughts, emotions, body sensations—anything that stands out.)

_____

_____

_____

Mood

How do you feel right now?
(Circle the one that represents how you feel.)

Energy Level

(Just notice— this isn't about motivation.)

How do I want to feel today?
(Write a word or phrase, or circle one.)

CALM • LIGHTER • STEADY • CONFIDENT
SAFE • FOCUSED • MYSELF

_____

_____

Today's Affirmation or Intention

(Keep it simple. One sentence is enough.)

_____

_____

_____

Today, I give myself permission to take this one step at a time.

Evening Reflection

You made it through the day. That matters.

Mood
How did you feel overall today?

What challenged me today?
(Externally or internally—both count.)

_____

_____

_____

What helped me feel even a little stronger or lighter today? (Small things matter more than you think.)

_____

_____

One thing I'm grateful for today:
(It can be about yourself, someone else, or a quiet moment.)

_____

_____

_____

Gentle Reminder: *If today felt heavy, that doesn't mean you failed. It means you showed up—and that's enough for today.*

TODAY'S LETTING-GO PRACTICE: Act of Release

Today, practice the mirror talk exercise. Stand in front of a mirror, look yourself in the eye, take one deep breath, and say the week's mantra out loud: "I deserve my own compassion."

DAY 39

Morning Intention

Take a breath before you begin.

What am I noticing in myself this morning? (Thoughts, emotions, body sensations—anything that stands out.)

_____

_____

_____

Mood
How do you feel right now?
(Circle the one that represents how you feel.)

Energy Level
(Just notice—
this isn't about
motivation.)

How do I want to feel today?
(Write a word or phrase, or circle one.)

CALM • LIGHTER • STEADY • CONFIDENT
SAFE • FOCUSED • MYSELF

_____

_____

Today's Affirmation or Intention
(Keep it simple. One sentence is enough.)

_____

_____

_____

*Today, I give myself permission
to take this one step at a time.*

Evening Reflection

*You made it through the day.
That matters.*

Mood
How did you feel overall today?

What challenged me today?
(Externally or internally—both count.)

_____

_____

_____

What helped me feel even a little stronger or lighter today? (Small things matter more than you think.)

_____

_____

_____

One thing I'm grateful for today:
(It can be about yourself, someone else, or a quiet moment.)

_____

_____

_____

Gentle Reminder: *If today felt heavy, that doesn't mean you failed. It means you showed up—and that's enough for today.*

TODAY'S LETTING-GO PRACTICE: Mindful Detachment

Self-criticism often creates physical tension. When you notice a harsh inner voice today, scan your body. Are your shoulders tense? Is your jaw clenched? Notice the tension, then consciously soften that part of your body. Breathe into it and let it relax.

_____

_____

_____

_____

_____

_____

_____

DAY 40

Morning Intention

Take a breath before you begin.

What am I noticing in myself this morning? (Thoughts, emotions, body sensations—anything that stands out.)

_____

_____

_____

Mood
How do you feel right now?
(Circle the one that represents how you feel.)

Energy Level
(Just notice—this isn't about motivation.)

How do I want to feel today?
(Write a word or phrase, or circle one.)

CALM • LIGHTER • STEADY • CONFIDENT
SAFE • FOCUSED • MYSELF

_____

_____

Today's Affirmation or Intention
(Keep it simple. One sentence is enough.)

_____

_____

Today, I give myself permission to take this one step at a time.

Evening Reflection

You made it through the day. That matters.

Mood
How did you feel overall today?

What challenged me today?
(Externally or internally—both count.)

_____

_____

_____

What helped me feel even a little stronger or lighter today? (Small things matter more than you think.)

_____

_____

_____

One thing I'm grateful for today:
(It can be about yourself, someone else, or a quiet moment.)

_____

_____

_____

Gentle Reminder: *If today felt heavy, that doesn't mean you failed. It means you showed up—and that's enough for today.*

TODAY'S LETTING-GO PRACTICE:
Reclaim Your Peace (Boundaries)

Set a boundary against hopeless self-talk. If the thought "I'll never change" arises, gently but firmly replace it with, "I'm growing daily."

DAY 41

Morning Intention

Take a breath before you begin.

What am I noticing in myself this morning? (Thoughts, emotions, body sensations—anything that stands out.)

_____

_____

_____

Mood
How do you feel right now?
(Circle the one that represents how you feel.)

Energy Level
(Just notice—
this isn't about
motivation.)

How do I want to feel today?
(Write a word or phrase, or circle one.)

CALM • LIGHTER • STEADY • CONFIDENT
SAFE • FOCUSED • MYSELF

_____

_____

Today's Affirmation or Intention
(Keep it simple. One sentence is enough.)

_____

_____

_____

*Today, I give myself permission
to take this one step at a time.*

Evening Reflection

*You made it through the day.
That matters.*

Mood
How did you feel overall today?

What challenged me today?
(Externally or internally—both count.)

_____

_____

_____

What helped me feel even a little stronger or lighter today? (Small things matter more than you think.)

_____

_____

_____

One thing I'm grateful for today:
(It can be about yourself, someone else, or a quiet moment.)

_____

_____

Gentle Reminder: *If today felt heavy, that doesn't mean you failed. It means you showed up—and that's enough for today.*

TODAY'S LETTING-GO PRACTICE: Express and Externalize

Today's practice is to write a love note to yourself. It can be short. Acknowledge your effort on this journey and thank yourself for showing up.

_____

_____

_____

_____

_____

_____

_____

DAY 42

Morning Intention

Take a breath before you begin.

What am I noticing in myself this morning? (Thoughts, emotions, body sensations—anything that stands out.)

_____

_____

_____

Mood
How do you feel right now?
(Circle the one that represents how you feel.)

Energy Level
(Just notice—this isn't about motivation.)

How do I want to feel today?
(Write a word or phrase, or circle one.)

CALM • LIGHTER • STEADY • CONFIDENT
SAFE • FOCUSED • MYSELF

_____

_____

Today's Affirmation or Intention
(Keep it simple. One sentence is enough.)

_____

_____

_____

Today, I give myself permission to take this one step at a time.

Evening Reflection

You made it through the day. That matters.

Mood
How did you feel overall today?

What challenged me today?
(Externally or internally—both count.)

_____

_____

_____

What helped me feel even a little stronger or lighter today? (Small things matter more than you think.)

_____

_____

_____

One thing I'm grateful for today:
(It can be about yourself, someone else, or a quiet moment.)

_____

_____

_____

Gentle Reminder: *If today felt heavy, that doesn't mean you failed. It means you showed up—and that's enough for today.*

TODAY'S LETTING-GO PRACTICE: Notice the Lightness

This is your End-of-Week Reflection. What did you forgive yourself for this week? How did it feel to offer yourself even a small moment of the compassion you deserve?

_____

_____

_____

_____

_____

_____

_____

YOGA POSE: Legs Up the Wall

Calms nervous system, relieves tired legs, and stretches, offering a restorative practice for self-compassion.

BREATHWORK EXERCISE: Deep Diaphragmatic Breathing

Activates parasympathetic nervous system, reduces heart rate/ blood pressure, promotes relaxation, and improves lung capacity, fostering a deep sense of calm and self-acceptance.

See appendix at the back of the book for more details
on Yoga Poses and Breathwork Exercises.

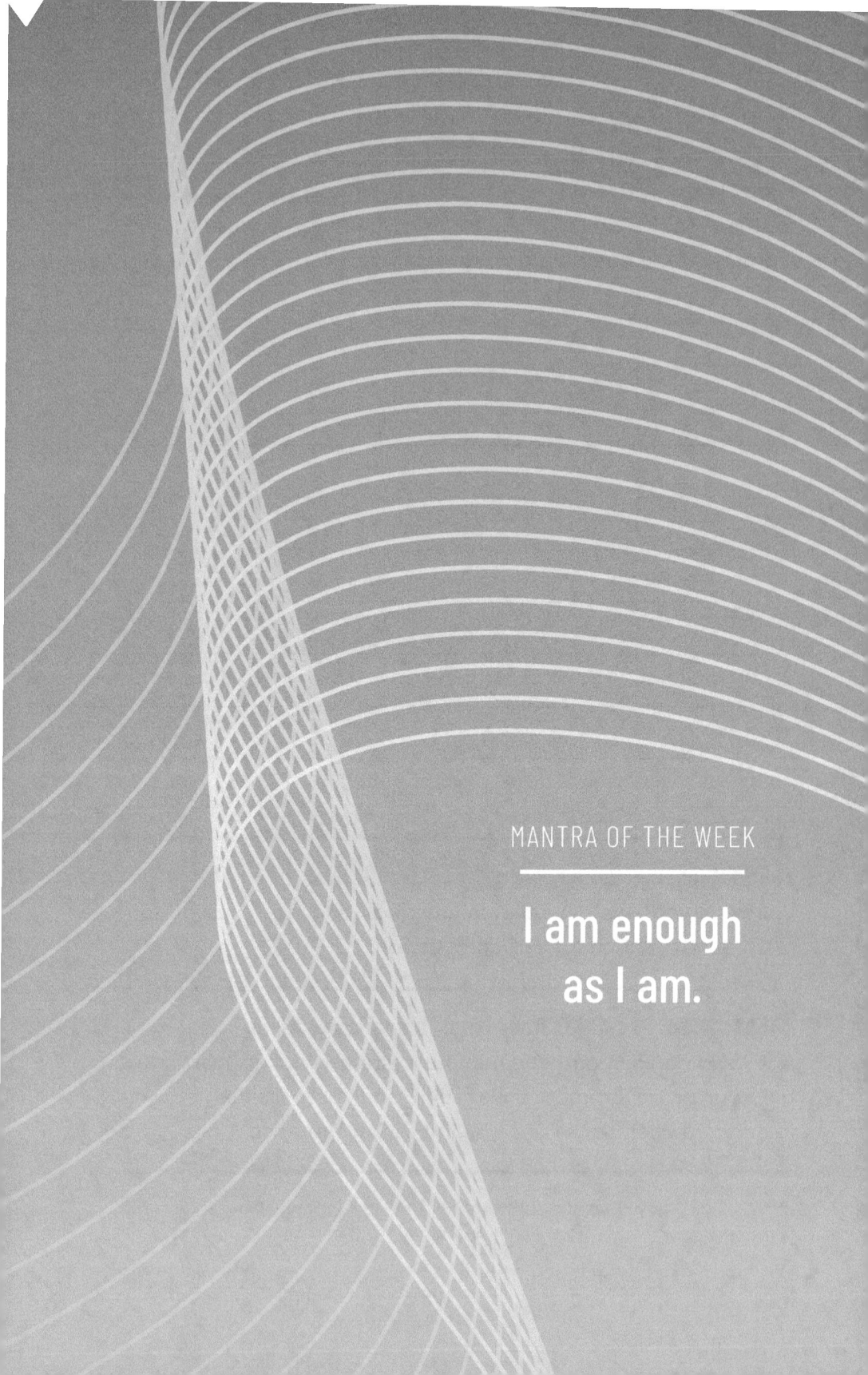

MANTRA OF THE WEEK

I am enough
as I am.

WEEK 7

Rebuilding
Confidence

DAY 43

Morning Intention

Take a breath before you begin.

What am I noticing in myself this morning? (Thoughts, emotions, body sensations—anything that stands out.)

_____

_____

_____

Mood
How do you feel right now?
(Circle the one that represents how you feel.)

Energy Level
(Just notice—
this isn't about
motivation.)

How do I want to feel today?
(Write a word or phrase, or circle one.)

CALM • LIGHTER • STEADY • CONFIDENT
SAFE • FOCUSED • MYSELF

_____

_____

Today's Affirmation or Intention
(Keep it simple. One sentence is enough.)

_____

_____

_____

*Today, I give myself permission
to take this one step at a time.*

Evening Reflection

*You made it through the day.
That matters.*

Mood
How did you feel overall today?

What challenged me today?
(Externally or internally—both count.)

_____

_____

_____

What helped me feel even a little stronger or lighter today? (Small things matter more than you think.)

_____

_____

_____

One thing I'm grateful for today:
(It can be about yourself, someone else, or a quiet moment.)

_____

_____

_____

Gentle Reminder: *If today felt heavy, that doesn't mean you failed. It means you showed up—and that's enough for today.*

TODAY'S LETTING-GO PRACTICE: Identify the Burden

The burden this week is a specific insecurity. Where in your life do you feel "not enough"? Identify one area of comparison or self-doubt that you are ready to challenge.

_____

_____

_____

_____

_____

_____

_____

DAY 44

Morning Intention

Take a breath before you begin.

What am I noticing in myself this morning? (Thoughts, emotions, body sensations—anything that stands out.)

_____

_____

_____

Mood
How do you feel right now?
(Circle the one that represents how you feel.)

Energy Level
(Just notice—this isn't about motivation.)

How do I want to feel today?
(Write a word or phrase, or circle one.)

CALM • LIGHTER • STEADY • CONFIDENT
SAFE • FOCUSED • MYSELF

_____

_____

Today's Affirmation or Intention
(Keep it simple. One sentence is enough.)

_____

_____

_____

Today, I give myself permission to take this one step at a time.

Evening Reflection

You made it through the day. That matters.

Mood
How did you feel overall today?

What challenged me today?
(Externally or internally—both count.)

_____

_____

_____

What helped me feel even a little stronger or lighter today? (Small things matter more than you think.)

_____

_____

_____

One thing I'm grateful for today:
(It can be about yourself, someone else, or a quiet moment.)

_____

_____

_____

Gentle Reminder: *If today felt heavy, that doesn't mean you failed. It means you showed up—and that's enough for today.*

TODAY'S LETTING-GO PRACTICE: Write to Understand

List three things you do well. They don't have to be grand accomplishments. Maybe you make a great cup of coffee, are a good listener, or are skilled at a particular hobby. Focus on your strengths.

_____

_____

_____

_____

_____

_____

_____

DAY 45

Morning Intention

Take a breath before you begin.

What am I noticing in myself this morning? (Thoughts, emotions, body sensations—anything that stands out.)

_____

_____

_____

Mood
How do you feel right now?
(Circle the one that represents how you feel.)

Energy Level
(Just notice—this isn't about motivation.)

How do I want to feel today?
(Write a word or phrase, or circle one.)

CALM • LIGHTER • STEADY • CONFIDENT
SAFE • FOCUSED • MYSELF

_____

_____

Today's Affirmation or Intention
(Keep it simple. One sentence is enough.)

_____

_____

_____

Today, I give myself permission to take this one step at a time.

Evening Reflection

*You made it through the day.
That matters.*

Mood
How did you feel overall today?

What challenged me today?
(Externally or internally—both count.)

_____

_____

_____

What helped me feel even a little stronger or lighter today? (Small things matter more than you think.)

_____

_____

_____

One thing I'm grateful for today:
(It can be about yourself, someone else, or a quiet moment.)

_____

_____

_____

Gentle Reminder: *If today felt heavy, that doesn't mean you failed. It means you showed up—and that's enough for today.*

TODAY'S LETTING-GO PRACTICE: Act of Release

Stand up, plant your feet firmly, and hold a confident posture for 60 seconds (e.g., hands on hips, or chest out and head held high). While holding the pose, repeat this week's mantra, "I am enough as I am," either silently or aloud.

DAY 46

Morning Intention

Take a breath before you begin.

What am I noticing in myself this morning? (Thoughts, emotions, body sensations—anything that stands out.)

_____

_____

_____

Mood
How do you feel right now?
(Circle the one that represents how you feel.)

Energy Level
(Just notice—this isn't about motivation.)

How do I want to feel today?
(Write a word or phrase, or circle one.)

CALM • LIGHTER • STEADY • CONFIDENT
SAFE • FOCUSED • MYSELF

_____

_____

Today's Affirmation or Intention
(Keep it simple. One sentence is enough.)

_____

_____

_____

Today, I give myself permission to take this one step at a time.

Evening Reflection

You made it through the day. That matters.

Mood
How did you feel overall today?

What challenged me today?
(Externally or internally—both count.)

_____

_____

_____

What helped me feel even a little stronger or lighter today? (Small things matter more than you think.)

_____

_____

_____

One thing I'm grateful for today:
(It can be about yourself, someone else, or a quiet moment.)

_____

_____

_____

Gentle Reminder: *If today felt heavy, that doesn't mean you failed. It means you showed up—and that's enough for today.*

TODAY'S LETTING-GO PRACTICE: Mindful Detachment

The mind often compares itself to others. When you notice a thought of comparison arise today, simply label it in your mind as "comparing." You don't need to fight it. Just notice it, label it, and let it drift by without giving it more energy.

DAY 47

Morning Intention

Take a breath before you begin.

What am I noticing in myself this morning? (Thoughts, emotions, body sensations—anything that stands out.)

_____

_____

_____

Mood
How do you feel right now?
(Circle the one that represents how you feel.)

Energy Level
(Just notice—this isn't about motivation.)

How do I want to feel today?
(Write a word or phrase, or circle one.)

CALM • LIGHTER • STEADY • CONFIDENT
SAFE • FOCUSED • MYSELF

_____

_____

Today's Affirmation or Intention
(Keep it simple. One sentence is enough.)

_____

_____

_____

Today, I give myself permission to take this one step at a time.

Evening Reflection

You made it through the day. That matters.

Mood
How did you feel overall today?

What challenged me today?
(Externally or internally—both count.)

_____

_____

_____

What helped me feel even a little stronger or lighter today? (Small things matter more than you think.)

_____

_____

_____

One thing I'm grateful for today:
(It can be about yourself, someone else, or a quiet moment.)

_____

_____

_____

Gentle Reminder: *If today felt heavy, that doesn't mean you failed. It means you showed up—and that's enough for today.*

TODAY'S LETTING-GO PRACTICE:
Reclaim Your Peace (Boundaries)

Your boundary today is against comparison thoughts. When you catch yourself comparing, gently stop the thought and replace it with a self-affirmation. For example, "Her path is not my path. I am proud of where I am."

DAY 48

Morning Intention

Take a breath before you begin.

What am I noticing in myself this morning? (Thoughts, emotions, body sensations—anything that stands out.)

_____

_____

_____

Mood
How do you feel right now?
(Circle the one that represents how you feel.)

Energy Level
(Just notice—this isn't about motivation.)

How do I want to feel today?
(Write a word or phrase, or circle one.)

CALM • LIGHTER • STEADY • CONFIDENT
SAFE • FOCUSED • MYSELF

_____

_____

Today's Affirmation or Intention
(Keep it simple. One sentence is enough.)

_____

_____

Today, I give myself permission to take this one step at a time.

Evening Reflection

You made it through the day. That matters.

Mood
How did you feel overall today?

What challenged me today?
(Externally or internally—both count.)

_____

_____

_____

What helped me feel even a little stronger or lighter today? (Small things matter more than you think.)

_____

_____

_____

One thing I'm grateful for today:
(It can be about yourself, someone else, or a quiet moment.)

_____

_____

_____

Gentle Reminder: *If today felt heavy, that doesn't mean you failed. It means you showed up—and that's enough for today.*

TODAY'S LETTING-GO PRACTICE: Express and Externalize

Today's practice is affirmation art. Write this week's mantra "I am enough as I am" on a piece of paper. Decorate the page with colors, doodles, or images that make you feel strong and confident.

DAY 49

Morning Intention

Take a breath before you begin.

What am I noticing in myself this morning? (Thoughts, emotions, body sensations—anything that stands out.)

_____

_____

_____

Mood

How do you feel right now?
(Circle the one that represents how you feel.)

Energy Level

(Just notice—
this isn't about
motivation.)

How do I want to feel today?
(Write a word or phrase, or circle one.)

CALM • LIGHTER • STEADY • CONFIDENT
SAFE • FOCUSED • MYSELF

_____

_____

Today's Affirmation or Intention
(Keep it simple. One sentence is enough.)

_____

_____

_____

*Today, I give myself permission
to take this one step at a time.*

Evening Reflection

*You made it through the day.
That matters.*

Mood
How did you feel overall today?

What challenged me today?
(Externally or internally—both count.)

_____

_____

_____

What helped me feel even a little stronger or lighter today? (Small things matter more than you think.)

_____

_____

_____

One thing I'm grateful for today:
(It can be about yourself, someone else, or a quiet moment.)

_____

_____

_____

Gentle Reminder: *If today felt heavy, that doesn't mean you failed. It means you showed up—and that's enough for today.*

TODAY'S LETTING-GO PRACTICE: Notice the Lightness

This is your End-of-Week Reflection. Look back at the three things you do well from Day 44. What new strength did you notice in yourself this week? Acknowledge the feeling of being "enough," even for a moment.

_____

_____

_____

_____

_____

_____

_____

YOGA POSE: Bridge Pose

Strengthens back/glutes/hamstrings, opens chest, calms brain, and alleviates stress, promoting a sense of inner strength and openness.

BREATHWORK EXERCISE: Humming Bee Breath

Calms nerves, reduces stress/anxiety, improves focus, and aids sleep, supporting a steady and focused approach to rebuilding confidence.

See appendix at the back of the book for more details
on Yoga Poses and Breathwork Exercises.

"No" is a
complete sentence.

Boundaries and Protection

DAY 50

Morning Intention

Take a breath before you begin.

What am I noticing in myself this morning? (Thoughts, emotions, body sensations—anything that stands out.)

_____

_____

_____

Mood
How do you feel right now?
(Circle the one that represents how you feel.)

Energy Level
(Just notice—this isn't about motivation.)

How do I want to feel today?
(Write a word or phrase, or circle one.)

CALM • LIGHTER • STEADY • CONFIDENT
SAFE • FOCUSED • MYSELF

_____

_____

Today's Affirmation or Intention
(Keep it simple. One sentence is enough.)

_____

_____

_____

Today, I give myself permission to take this one step at a time.

Evening Reflection

You made it through the day. That matters.

Mood
How did you feel overall today?

What challenged me today?
(Externally or internally—both count.)

_____

_____

_____

What helped me feel even a little stronger or lighter today? (Small things matter more than you think.)

_____

_____

_____

One thing I'm grateful for today:
(It can be about yourself, someone else, or a quiet moment.)

_____

_____

_____

Gentle Reminder: *If today felt heavy, that doesn't mean you failed. It means you showed up—and that's enough for today.*

TODAY'S LETTING-GO PRACTICE: Identify the Burden

The burden this week is an energy leak. Identify one area in your life—a relationship, a task, or a habit—where you feel your energy is being drained because a boundary is weak or missing.

_____

_____

_____

_____

_____

_____

_____

DAY 51

Morning Intention

Take a breath before you begin.

What am I noticing in myself this morning? (Thoughts, emotions, body sensations—anything that stands out.)

_____

_____

_____

Mood
How do you feel right now?
(Circle the one that represents how you feel.)

Energy Level
(Just notice—this isn't about motivation.)

How do I want to feel today?
(Write a word or phrase, or circle one.)

CALM • LIGHTER • STEADY • CONFIDENT
SAFE • FOCUSED • MYSELF

_____

_____

Today's Affirmation or Intention
(Keep it simple. One sentence is enough.)

_____

_____

_____

Today, I give myself permission to take this one step at a time.

Evening Reflection

You made it through the day. That matters.

Mood
How did you feel overall today?

What challenged me today?
(Externally or internally—both count.)

_____

_____

_____

What helped me feel even a little stronger or lighter today? (Small things matter more than you think.)

_____

_____

_____

One thing I'm grateful for today:
(It can be about yourself, someone else, or a quiet moment.)

_____

_____

_____

Gentle Reminder: *If today felt heavy, that doesn't mean you failed. It means you showed up—and that's enough for today.*

TODAY'S LETTING-GO PRACTICE: Write to Understand

Write about the situation you identified yesterday. What fears or people-pleasing thoughts make it difficult to set a boundary there? What would you gain (peace, time, energy) if a healthy boundary were in place?

_____

_____

_____

_____

_____

_____

_____

_____

DAY 52

Morning Intention

Take a breath before you begin.

What am I noticing in myself this morning? (Thoughts, emotions, body sensations—anything that stands out.)

_____

_____

_____

Mood
How do you feel right now?
(Circle the one that represents how you feel.)

Energy Level
(Just notice— this isn't about motivation.)

How do I want to feel today?
(Write a word or phrase, or circle one.)

CALM • LIGHTER • STEADY • CONFIDENT
SAFE • FOCUSED • MYSELF

_____

_____

Today's Affirmation or Intention
(Keep it simple. One sentence is enough.)

_____

_____

_____

Today, I give myself permission to take this one step at a time.

Evening Reflection

You made it through the day. That matters.

Mood
How did you feel overall today?

What challenged me today?
(Externally or internally—both count.)

_____

_____

_____

What helped me feel even a little stronger or lighter today? (Small things matter more than you think.)

_____

_____

_____

One thing I'm grateful for today:
(It can be about yourself, someone else, or a quiet moment.)

_____

_____

_____

Gentle Reminder: *If today felt heavy, that doesn't mean you failed. It means you showed up—and that's enough for today.*

TODAY'S LETTING-GO PRACTICE: Act of Release

Find a private space and practice the physical act of saying "no." Say it out loud three times: once softly, once in a normal tone, and once with firmness. The goal is to become comfortable with the word itself, separate from any guilt.

DAY 53

Morning Intention

Take a breath before you begin.

What am I noticing in myself this morning? (Thoughts, emotions, body sensations—anything that stands out.)

_____

_____

_____

Mood
How do you feel right now?
(Circle the one that represents how you feel.)

Energy Level
(Just notice— this isn't about motivation.)

How do I want to feel today?
(Write a word or phrase, or circle one.)

CALM • LIGHTER • STEADY • CONFIDENT
SAFE • FOCUSED • MYSELF

_____

_____

Today's Affirmation or Intention
(Keep it simple. One sentence is enough.)

_____

_____

_____

Today, I give myself permission to take this one step at a time.

Evening Reflection

*You made it through the day.
That matters.*

Mood
How did you feel overall today?

What challenged me today?
(Externally or internally—both count.)

_____

_____

_____

What helped me feel even a little stronger or lighter today? (Small things matter more than you think.)

_____

_____

_____

One thing I'm grateful for today:
(It can be about yourself, someone else, or a quiet moment.)

_____

_____

_____

Gentle Reminder: *If today felt heavy, that doesn't mean you failed. It means you showed up—and that's enough for today.*

TODAY'S LETTING-GO PRACTICE: Mindful Detachment

When you think about setting the boundary you need, notice any feelings of guilt or anxiety that arise. Acknowledge the feeling without judgment. Label it "the discomfort of growth" and recognize it as a sign of positive change, not a warning to stop.

DAY 54

Morning Intention

Take a breath before you begin.

What am I noticing in myself this morning? (Thoughts, emotions, body sensations—anything that stands out.)

_____

_____

_____

Mood
How do you feel right now?
(Circle the one that represents how you feel.)

Energy Level
(Just notice—this isn't about motivation.)

How do I want to feel today?
(Write a word or phrase, or circle one.)

CALM • LIGHTER • STEADY • CONFIDENT
SAFE • FOCUSED • MYSELF

_____

_____

Today's Affirmation or Intention
(Keep it simple. One sentence is enough.)

_____

_____

_____

Today, I give myself permission to take this one step at a time.

Evening Reflection

*You made it through the day.
That matters.*

Mood
How did you feel overall today?

What challenged me today?
(Externally or internally—both count.)

_____

_____

_____

What helped me feel even a little stronger or lighter today? (Small things matter more than you think.)

_____

_____

_____

One thing I'm grateful for today:
(It can be about yourself, someone else, or a quiet moment.)

_____

_____

_____

Gentle Reminder: *If today felt heavy, that doesn't mean you failed. It means you showed up—and that's enough for today.*

TODAY'S LETTING-GO PRACTICE:
Reclaim Your Peace (Boundaries)

Today's challenge is to say "no" once this week without guilt. This could be a small, gentle "no," such as "I can't make it," or "Not right now." The goal is to practice honoring your own capacity.

DAY 55

Morning Intention

Take a breath before you begin.

What am I noticing in myself this morning? (Thoughts, emotions, body sensations—anything that stands out.)

_____

_____

_____

Mood
How do you feel right now?
(Circle the one that represents how you feel.)

Energy Level
(Just notice—this isn't about motivation.)

How do I want to feel today?
(Write a word or phrase, or circle one.)

CALM • LIGHTER • STEADY • CONFIDENT
SAFE • FOCUSED • MYSELF

_____

_____

Today's Affirmation or Intention
(Keep it simple. One sentence is enough.)

_____

_____

_____

Today, I give myself permission to take this one step at a time.

Evening Reflection

*You made it through the day.
That matters.*

Mood
How did you feel overall today?

What challenged me today?
(Externally or internally—both count.)

_____

_____

_____

What helped me feel even a little stronger or lighter today? (Small things matter more than you think.)

_____

_____

_____

One thing I'm grateful for today:
(It can be about yourself, someone else, or a quiet moment.)

_____

_____

_____

Gentle Reminder: *If today felt heavy, that doesn't mean you failed. It means you showed up—and that's enough for today.*

TODAY'S LETTING-GO PRACTICE: Express and Externalize

Today, do the boundary building exercise. Draw a circle in the middle of the page and write "me" inside it. Around the circle, draw a protective barrier (a wall, a fence, a bubble). On the inside, write what you are protecting (e.g., your peace, your energy). On the outside, write what you are protecting it from.

DAY 56

Morning Intention

Take a breath before you begin.

What am I noticing in myself this morning? (Thoughts, emotions, body sensations—anything that stands out.)

_____

_____

_____

Mood
How do you feel right now?
(Circle the one that represents how you feel.)

Energy Level
(Just notice—this isn't about motivation.)

How do I want to feel today?
(Write a word or phrase, or circle one.)

CALM • LIGHTER • STEADY • CONFIDENT
SAFE • FOCUSED • MYSELF

_____

_____

Today's Affirmation or Intention
(Keep it simple. One sentence is enough.)

_____

_____

_____

Today, I give myself permission to take this one step at a time.

Evening Reflection

You made it through the day. That matters.

Mood
How did you feel overall today?

What challenged me today?
(Externally or internally—both count.)

_____

_____

_____

What helped me feel even a little stronger or lighter today? (Small things matter more than you think.)

_____

_____

_____

One thing I'm grateful for today:
(It can be about yourself, someone else, or a quiet moment.)

_____

_____

_____

Gentle Reminder: *If today felt heavy, that doesn't mean you failed. It means you showed up—and that's enough for today.*

TODAY'S LETTING-GO PRACTICE: Notice the Lightness

This is your End-of-Week Reflection. Where did you protect your energy this week? How did it feel to say "no" or reinforce a boundary, even in a small way? Acknowledge the self-respect in that action.

_____

_____

_____

_____

_____

_____

_____

_____

YOGA POSE: Downward-Facing Dog

Stretches whole body, strengthens arms/legs, calms brain, and relieves stress, providing a grounding and strengthening pose for establishing boundaries.

BREATHWORK EXERCISE: Box Breathing

Calms nerves, reduces stress, and improves focus/clarity, which can be helpful in maintaining resolve and clarity when setting boundaries.

See appendix at the back of the book for more details
on Yoga Poses and Breathwork Exercises.

REFLECTION ON THE PAST 4 WEEKS

What was your biggest insight or breakthrough during the last four weeks?

_____

_____

_____

_____

_____

_____

_____

What challenge did you face, and how did you overcome it (or what did you learn from it)?

_____

_____

_____

_____

_____

_____

_____

REFLECTION ON THE PAST 4 WEEKS

What is one thing you are grateful for from these past four weeks?

_____

_____

_____

_____

_____

_____

_____

How has your sense of peace or understanding of "letting go" evolved?

_____

_____

_____

_____

_____

_____

_____

_____

Gratitude turns pain into power.

Gratitude and Growth

DAY 57

Morning Intention	Evening Reflection

Take a breath before you begin.

You made it through the day. That matters.

What am I noticing in myself this morning? (Thoughts, emotions, body sensations—anything that stands out.)

_____

_____

_____

Mood
How did you feel overall today?

What challenged me today?
(Externally or internally—both count.)

_____

_____

_____

Mood
How do you feel right now?
(Circle the one that represents how you feel.)

Energy Level
(Just notice— this isn't about motivation.)

What helped me feel even a little stronger or lighter today? (Small things matter more than you think.)

_____

_____

_____

How do I want to feel today?
(Write a word or phrase, or circle one.)

CALM • LIGHTER • STEADY • CONFIDENT
SAFE • FOCUSED • MYSELF

_____

_____

Today's Affirmation or Intention
(Keep it simple. One sentence is enough.)

_____

_____

_____

One thing I'm grateful for today:
(It can be about yourself, someone else, or a quiet moment.)

_____

_____

_____

Today, I give myself permission to take this one step at a time.

Gentle Reminder: *If today felt heavy, that doesn't mean you failed. It means you showed up—and that's enough for today.*

TODAY'S LETTING-GO PRACTICE: Identify the Burden

The burden this week is a feeling of lack. Identify one area in your life where you feel something is missing or not enough (e.g., lack of progress, time, or connection). This will be your focus for the week.

_____

_____

_____

_____

_____

_____

_____

DAY 58

Morning Intention

Take a breath before you begin.

What am I noticing in myself this morning? (Thoughts, emotions, body sensations—anything that stands out.)

_____

_____

_____

Mood
How do you feel right now?
(Circle the one that represents how you feel.)

Energy Level
(Just notice—this isn't about motivation.)

How do I want to feel today?
(Write a word or phrase, or circle one.)

CALM • LIGHTER • STEADY • CONFIDENT
SAFE • FOCUSED • MYSELF

_____

_____

Today's Affirmation or Intention
(Keep it simple. One sentence is enough.)

_____

_____

_____

Today, I give myself permission to take this one step at a time.

Evening Reflection

You made it through the day. That matters.

Mood
How did you feel overall today?

What challenged me today?
(Externally or internally—both count.)

_____

_____

_____

What helped me feel even a little stronger or lighter today? (Small things matter more than you think.)

_____

_____

_____

One thing I'm grateful for today:
(It can be about yourself, someone else, or a quiet moment.)

_____

_____

_____

Gentle Reminder: *If today felt heavy, that doesn't mean you failed. It means you showed up—and that's enough for today.*

TODAY'S LETTING-GO PRACTICE: Write to Understand

Write about the feeling of lack you identified. Then, challenge that feeling by writing down three small pieces of evidence to the contrary. For example, if you feel a lack of progress, list three tiny steps you *have* taken.

_____

_____

_____

_____

_____

_____

_____

_____

DAY 59

Morning Intention

Take a breath before you begin.

What am I noticing in myself this morning? (Thoughts, emotions, body sensations—anything that stands out.)

_____

_____

_____

Mood
How do you feel right now?
(Circle the one that represents how you feel.)

Energy Level
(Just notice—
this isn't about
motivation.)

How do I want to feel today?
(Write a word or phrase, or circle one.)

CALM • LIGHTER • STEADY • CONFIDENT
SAFE • FOCUSED • MYSELF

_____

_____

Today's Affirmation or Intention
(Keep it simple. One sentence is enough.)

_____

_____

_____

*Today, I give myself permission
to take this one step at a time.*

Evening Reflection

*You made it through the day.
That matters.*

Mood
How did you feel overall today?

What challenged me today?
(Externally or internally—both count.)

_____

_____

_____

What helped me feel even a little stronger or lighter today? (Small things matter more than you think.)

_____

_____

_____

One thing I'm grateful for today:
(It can be about yourself, someone else, or a quiet moment.)

_____

_____

_____

Gentle Reminder: *If today felt heavy, that doesn't mean you failed. It means you showed up—and that's enough for today.*

TODAY'S LETTING-GO PRACTICE: Act of Release

Today, go on a gratitude hunt. Take a five-minute walk or simply look around your current space. Your only task is to find and physically point to three things you are grateful for but usually overlook (e.g., a comfortable chair, a favorite mug, the color of the sky).

_____

_____

_____

_____

_____

_____

_____

_____

DAY 60

Morning Intention

Take a breath before you begin.

What am I noticing in myself this morning? (Thoughts, emotions, body sensations—anything that stands out.)

_____

_____

_____

Mood
How do you feel right now?
(Circle the one that represents how you feel.)

Energy Level
(Just notice—this isn't about motivation.)

How do I want to feel today?
(Write a word or phrase, or circle one.)

CALM • LIGHTER • STEADY • CONFIDENT
SAFE • FOCUSED • MYSELF

_____

_____

Today's Affirmation or Intention
(Keep it simple. One sentence is enough.)

_____

_____

_____

Today, I give myself permission to take this one step at a time.

Evening Reflection

You made it through the day. That matters.

Mood
How did you feel overall today?

What challenged me today?
(Externally or internally—both count.)

_____

_____

_____

What helped me feel even a little stronger or lighter today? (Small things matter more than you think.)

_____

_____

_____

One thing I'm grateful for today:
(It can be about yourself, someone else, or a quiet moment.)

_____

_____

_____

Gentle Reminder: *If today felt heavy, that doesn't mean you failed. It means you showed up—and that's enough for today.*

TODAY'S LETTING-GO PRACTICE: Mindful Detachment

When a thought of scarcity or "not enough" arises, notice how that feeling manifests in your body. Does it feel like a tightness in your chest? A pit in your stomach? Observe the physical sensation with curiosity, creating a space between the feeling and your reaction to it.

_____

_____

_____

_____

_____

_____

_____

DAY 61

Morning Intention

Take a breath before you begin.

What am I noticing in myself this morning? (Thoughts, emotions, body sensations—anything that stands out.)

_____

_____

_____

Mood
How do you feel right now?
(Circle the one that represents how you feel.)

Energy Level
(Just notice— this isn't about motivation.)

How do I want to feel today?
(Write a word or phrase, or circle one.)

CALM • LIGHTER • STEADY • CONFIDENT
SAFE • FOCUSED • MYSELF

_____

_____

Today's Affirmation or Intention
(Keep it simple. One sentence is enough.)

_____

_____

_____

Today, I give myself permission to take this one step at a time.

Evening Reflection

You made it through the day. That matters.

Mood
How did you feel overall today?

What challenged me today?
(Externally or internally—both count.)

_____

_____

_____

What helped me feel even a little stronger or lighter today? (Small things matter more than you think.)

_____

_____

_____

One thing I'm grateful for today:
(It can be about yourself, someone else, or a quiet moment.)

_____

_____

_____

Gentle Reminder: *If today felt heavy, that doesn't mean you failed. It means you showed up—and that's enough for today.*

TODAY'S LETTING-GO PRACTICE:
Reclaim Your Peace (Boundaries)

Set a boundary against a lack mindset. When you notice a thought of lack today, challenge it by finding one small thing to appreciate in that exact moment. For example, if you think, "I don't have enough time," counter it with, "I am grateful for these five minutes I have right now."

DAY 62

Morning Intention

Take a breath before you begin.

What am I noticing in myself this morning? (Thoughts, emotions, body sensations—anything that stands out.)

_____

_____

_____

Mood
How do you feel right now?
(Circle the one that represents how you feel.)

Energy Level
(Just notice—this isn't about motivation.)

How do I want to feel today?
(Write a word or phrase, or circle one.)

CALM • LIGHTER • STEADY • CONFIDENT
SAFE • FOCUSED • MYSELF

_____

_____

Today's Affirmation or Intention
(Keep it simple. One sentence is enough.)

_____

_____

_____

Today, I give myself permission to take this one step at a time.

Evening Reflection

You made it through the day. That matters.

Mood
How did you feel overall today?

What challenged me today?
(Externally or internally—both count.)

_____

_____

_____

What helped me feel even a little stronger or lighter today? (Small things matter more than you think.)

_____

_____

_____

One thing I'm grateful for today:
(It can be about yourself, someone else, or a quiet moment.)

_____

_____

_____

Gentle Reminder: *If today felt heavy, that doesn't mean you failed. It means you showed up—and that's enough for today.*

TODAY'S LETTING-GO PRACTICE: Express and Externalize

Think about your journey so far. Find an object in your home that represents growth to you (e.g., a plant, a repaired item, a book you've read). Place it somewhere you can see it today as a physical reminder of your own resilience and progress.

_____

_____

_____

_____

_____

_____

_____

DAY 63

Morning Intention

Take a breath before you begin.

What am I noticing in myself this morning? (Thoughts, emotions, body sensations—anything that stands out.)

_____

_____

_____

Mood

How do you feel right now?
(Circle the one that represents how you feel.)

Energy Level

(Just notice— this isn't about motivation.)

How do I want to feel today?
(Write a word or phrase, or circle one.)

CALM • LIGHTER • STEADY • CONFIDENT
SAFE • FOCUSED • MYSELF

_____

_____

Today's Affirmation or Intention

(Keep it simple. One sentence is enough.)

_____

_____

_____

Today, I give myself permission to take this one step at a time.

Evening Reflection

You made it through the day. That matters.

Mood
How did you feel overall today?

What challenged me today?
(Externally or internally—both count.)

_____

_____

_____

What helped me feel even a little stronger or lighter today? (Small things matter more than you think.)

_____

_____

_____

One thing I'm grateful for today:
(It can be about yourself, someone else, or a quiet moment.)

_____

_____

_____

Gentle Reminder: *If today felt heavy, that doesn't mean you failed. It means you showed up—and that's enough for today.*

TODAY'S LETTING-GO PRACTICE: Notice the Lightness

This is your End-of-Week Reflection. What did gratitude shift in you this week? Look back at your Evening Reflections. What did focusing on gratitude and growth, instead of lack, change for you?

_____

_____

_____

_____

_____

_____

_____

_____

YOGA POSE: Easy Pose

Promotes calmness/mental clarity, ideal for meditation/breathwork, creating a peaceful space for cultivating gratitude.

BREATHWORK EXERCISE: Resonant Breathing

Balances nervous system, promotes relaxation, and reduces stress, fostering a sense of harmony and openness to growth.

See appendix at the back of the book for more details
on Yoga Poses and Breathwork Exercises.

MANTRA OF THE WEEK

I am building
a life I love.

Creating
a Vision

DAY 64

Morning Intention

Take a breath before you begin.

What am I noticing in myself this morning? (Thoughts, emotions, body sensations—anything that stands out.)

_____

_____

_____

Mood
How do you feel right now?
(Circle the one that represents how you feel.)

Energy Level
(Just notice—this isn't about motivation.)

How do I want to feel today?
(Write a word or phrase, or circle one.)

CALM • LIGHTER • STEADY • CONFIDENT
SAFE • FOCUSED • MYSELF

_____

_____

Today's Affirmation or Intention
(Keep it simple. One sentence is enough.)

_____

_____

_____

Today, I give myself permission to take this one step at a time.

Evening Reflection

You made it through the day. That matters.

Mood
How did you feel overall today?

What challenged me today?
(Externally or internally—both count.)

_____

_____

_____

What helped me feel even a little stronger or lighter today? (Small things matter more than you think.)

_____

_____

_____

One thing I'm grateful for today:
(It can be about yourself, someone else, or a quiet moment.)

_____

_____

_____

Gentle Reminder: *If today felt heavy, that doesn't mean you failed. It means you showed up—and that's enough for today.*

TODAY'S LETTING-GO PRACTICE: Identify the Burden

The burden this week is hopelessness, or the feeling of being stuck.
Identify one area of your life where it feels difficult to imagine
a positive future. This is the area you will bring a new vision to
this week.

_____

_____

_____

_____

_____

_____

_____

DAY 65

Morning Intention

Take a breath before you begin.

What am I noticing in myself this morning? (Thoughts, emotions, body sensations—anything that stands out.)

_____

_____

_____

Mood
How do you feel right now?
(Circle the one that represents how you feel.)

Energy Level
(Just notice—this isn't about motivation.)

How do I want to feel today?
(Write a word or phrase, or circle one.)

CALM • LIGHTER • STEADY • CONFIDENT
SAFE • FOCUSED • MYSELF

_____

_____

Today's Affirmation or Intention
(Keep it simple. One sentence is enough.)

_____

_____

_____

Today, I give myself permission to take this one step at a time.

Evening Reflection

You made it through the day. That matters.

Mood
How did you feel overall today?

What challenged me today?
(Externally or internally—both count.)

_____

_____

_____

What helped me feel even a little stronger or lighter today? (Small things matter more than you think.)

_____

_____

_____

One thing I'm grateful for today:
(It can be about yourself, someone else, or a quiet moment.)

_____

_____

_____

Gentle Reminder: *If today felt heavy, that doesn't mean you failed. It means you showed up—and that's enough for today.*

TODAY'S LETTING-GO PRACTICE: Write to Understand

Visualize your best possible day and write it out in detail. What would you do? Who would you see? How would you feel from morning to night? Don't worry about how it could happen; just focus on the "what."

DAY 66

Morning Intention

Take a breath before you begin.

What am I noticing in myself this morning? (Thoughts, emotions, body sensations—anything that stands out.)

_____

_____

_____

Mood
How do you feel right now?
(Circle the one that represents how you feel.)

Energy Level
(Just notice—this isn't about motivation.)

How do I want to feel today?
(Write a word or phrase, or circle one.)

CALM • LIGHTER • STEADY • CONFIDENT
SAFE • FOCUSED • MYSELF

_____

_____

Today's Affirmation or Intention
(Keep it simple. One sentence is enough.)

_____

_____

_____

Today, I give myself permission to take this one step at a time.

Evening Reflection

You made it through the day.
That matters.

Mood
How did you feel overall today?

What challenged me today?
(Externally or internally—both count.)

_____

_____

_____

What helped me feel even a little stronger or lighter today? (Small things matter more than you think.)

_____

_____

_____

One thing I'm grateful for today:
(It can be about yourself, someone else, or a quiet moment.)

_____

_____

Gentle Reminder: *If today felt heavy, that doesn't mean you failed. It means you showed up—and that's enough for today.*

TODAY'S LETTING-GO PRACTICE: Act of Release

Take one tiny, physical step toward the vision you wrote yesterday. If your vision includes peace, tidy one small corner of a room. If it includes health, do two minutes of stretching. The action connects your future dream to your present reality.

DAY 67

Morning Intention

Take a breath before you begin.

What am I noticing in myself this morning? (Thoughts, emotions, body sensations—anything that stands out.)

_____

_____

_____

Mood
How do you feel right now?
(Circle the one that represents how you feel.)

Energy Level
(Just notice—
this isn't about
motivation.)

How do I want to feel today?
(Write a word or phrase, or circle one.)

CALM • LIGHTER • STEADY • CONFIDENT
SAFE • FOCUSED • MYSELF

_____

_____

Today's Affirmation or Intention
(Keep it simple. One sentence is enough.)

_____

_____

_____

*Today, I give myself permission
to take this one step at a time.*

Evening Reflection

*You made it through the day.
That matters.*

Mood
How did you feel overall today?

What challenged me today?
(Externally or internally—both count.)

_____

_____

_____

What helped me feel even a little stronger or lighter today? (Small things matter more than you think.)

_____

_____

_____

One thing I'm grateful for today:
(It can be about yourself, someone else, or a quiet moment.)

_____

_____

_____

Gentle Reminder: *If today felt heavy, that doesn't mean you failed. It means you showed up—and that's enough for today.*

TODAY'S LETTING-GO PRACTICE: Mindful Detachment

When you think about your vision, you might hear a voice of doubt. Today, just notice that voice. When a thought like "That's impossible" appears, label it "doubting" and let it pass without argument, gently returning your focus to a positive part of your vision.

_____

_____

_____

_____

_____

_____

_____

_____

DAY 68

Morning Intention

Take a breath before you begin.

What am I noticing in myself this morning? (Thoughts, emotions, body sensations—anything that stands out.)

_____

_____

_____

Mood
How do you feel right now?
(Circle the one that represents how you feel.)

Energy Level
(Just notice—this isn't about motivation.)

How do I want to feel today?
(Write a word or phrase, or circle one.)

CALM • LIGHTER • STEADY • CONFIDENT
SAFE • FOCUSED • MYSELF

_____

_____

Today's Affirmation or Intention
(Keep it simple. One sentence is enough.)

_____

_____

_____

Today, I give myself permission to take this one step at a time.

Evening Reflection

You made it through the day. That matters.

Mood
How did you feel overall today?

What challenged me today?
(Externally or internally—both count.)

_____

_____

_____

What helped me feel even a little stronger or lighter today? (Small things matter more than you think.)

_____

_____

_____

One thing I'm grateful for today:
(It can be about yourself, someone else, or a quiet moment.)

_____

_____

_____

Gentle Reminder: *If today felt heavy, that doesn't mean you failed. It means you showed up—and that's enough for today.*

TODAY'S LETTING-GO PRACTICE:
Reclaim Your Peace (Boundaries)

Your boundary today is against hopelessness. If you have a hopeless thought, gently replace it with a thought of possibility. For example, instead of "Nothing will ever change," try "I am open to the possibility that things can be different."

DAY 69

Morning Intention

Take a breath before you begin.

What am I noticing in myself this morning? (Thoughts, emotions, body sensations—anything that stands out.)

_____

_____

_____

Mood
How do you feel right now?
(Circle the one that represents how you feel.)

Energy Level
(Just notice—
this isn't about
motivation.)

How do I want to feel today?
(Write a word or phrase, or circle one.)

CALM • LIGHTER • STEADY • CONFIDENT
SAFE • FOCUSED • MYSELF

_____

_____

Today's Affirmation or Intention
(Keep it simple. One sentence is enough.)

_____

_____

_____

*Today, I give myself permission
to take this one step at a time.*

Evening Reflection

*You made it through the day.
That matters.*

Mood
How did you feel overall today?

What challenged me today?
(Externally or internally—both count.)

_____

_____

_____

What helped me feel even a little stronger or lighter today? (Small things matter more than you think.)

_____

_____

_____

One thing I'm grateful for today:
(It can be about yourself, someone else, or a quiet moment.)

_____

_____

_____

Gentle Reminder: *If today felt heavy, that doesn't mean you failed. It means you showed up—and that's enough for today.*

TODAY'S LETTING-GO PRACTICE: Express and Externalize

Today's practice is a vision collage. Find or draw one single image that represents a key feeling of the life you are building. It could be a picture of a calm lake, a vibrant color, or a smiling face. Place it where you can see it.

DAY 70

Morning Intention	Evening Reflection

Morning Intention

Take a breath before you begin.

What am I noticing in myself this morning? (Thoughts, emotions, body sensations—anything that stands out.)

_____

_____

_____

Mood
How do you feel right now?
(Circle the one that represents how you feel.)

Energy Level
(Just notice—
this isn't about
motivation.)

How do I want to feel today?
(Write a word or phrase, or circle one.)

CALM • LIGHTER • STEADY • CONFIDENT
SAFE • FOCUSED • MYSELF

_____

_____

Today's Affirmation or Intention
(Keep it simple. One sentence is enough.)

_____

_____

_____

*Today, I give myself permission
to take this one step at a time.*

Evening Reflection

*You made it through the day.
That matters.*

Mood
How did you feel overall today?

What challenged me today?
(Externally or internally—both count.)

_____

_____

_____

What helped me feel even a little stronger or lighter today? (Small things matter more than you think.)

_____

_____

_____

One thing I'm grateful for today:
(It can be about yourself, someone else, or a quiet moment.)

_____

_____

Gentle Reminder: *If today felt heavy, that doesn't mean you failed. It means you showed up—and that's enough for today.*

TODAY'S LETTING-GO PRACTICE: Notice the Lightness

This is your End-of-Week Reflection. How did it feel to focus on a positive vision rather than a current problem? Did taking one small action make your desired future feel even a little more possible?

_____

_____

_____

_____

_____

_____

_____

YOGA POSE: Legs Up the Wall

Calms nervous system and promotes relaxation, ideal for quiet contemplation and visualizing a positive future.

BREATHWORK EXERCISE: Deep Diaphragmatic Breathing

Activates the parasympathetic nervous system and promotes deep relaxation, aiding in focused visualization and intention setting.

See appendix at the back of the book for more details
on Yoga Poses and Breathwork Exercises.

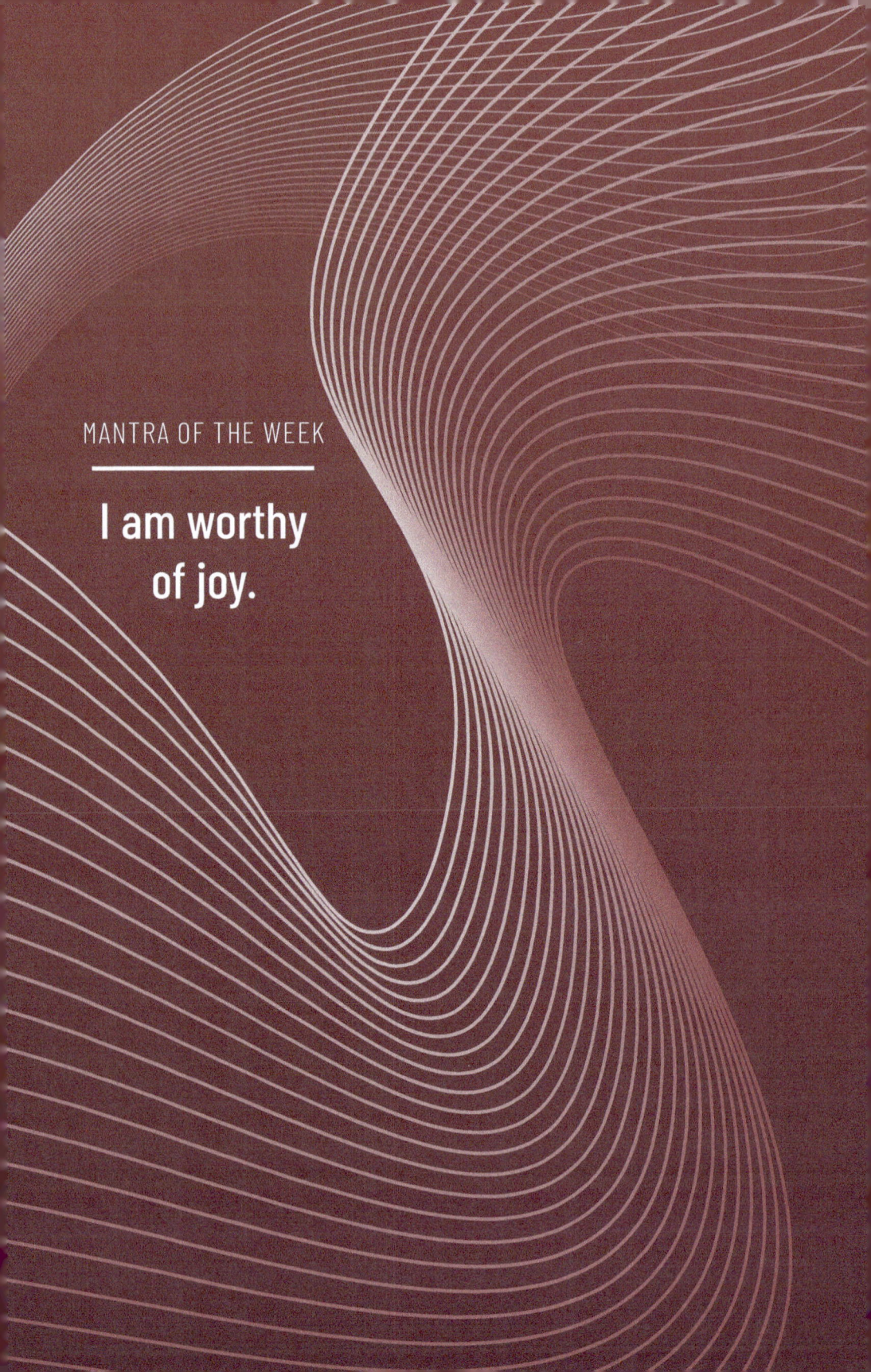

MANTRA OF THE WEEK
———

I am worthy of joy.

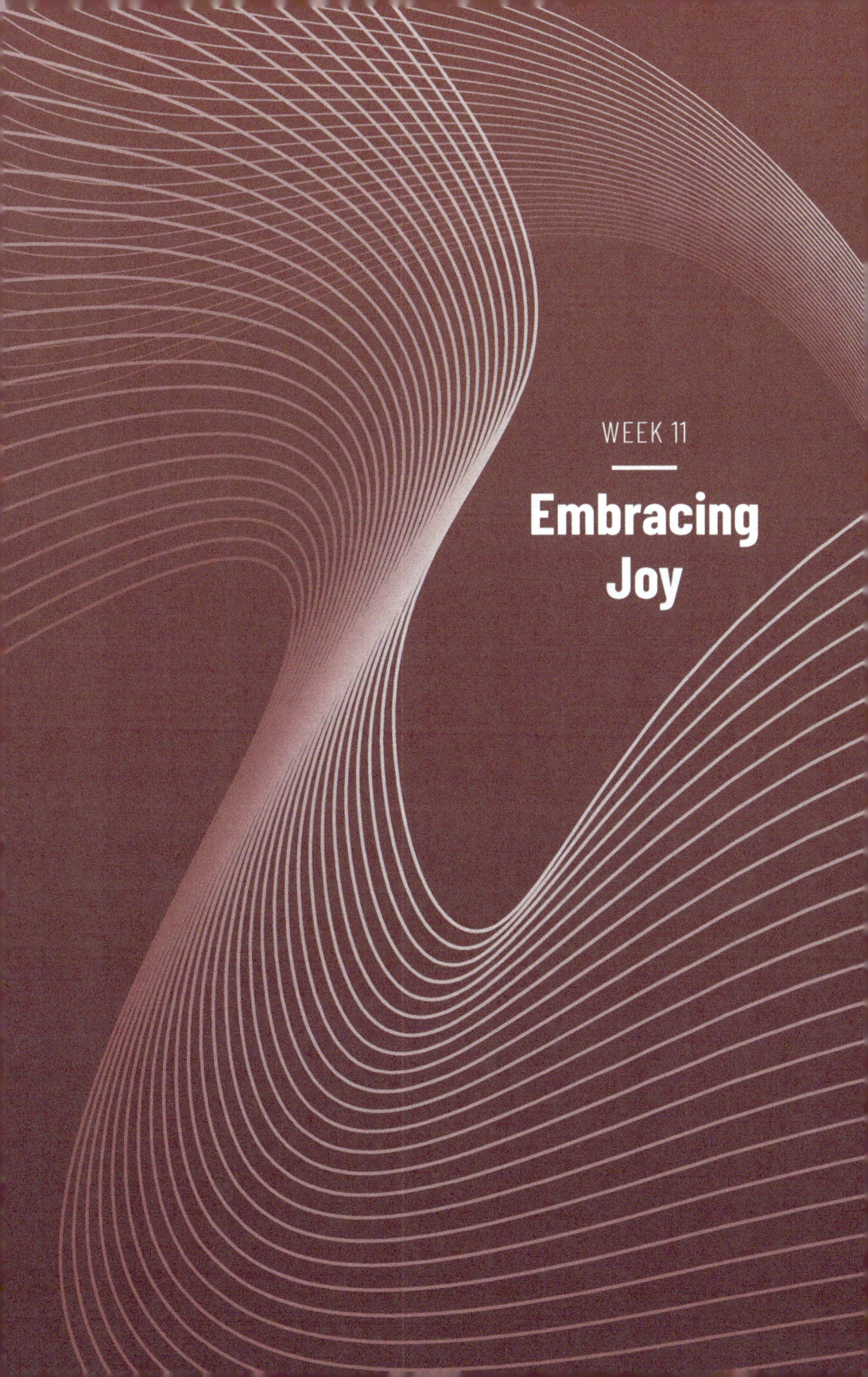

WEEK 11

Embracing Joy

DAY 71

Morning Intention

Take a breath before you begin.

What am I noticing in myself this morning? (Thoughts, emotions, body sensations—anything that stands out.)

_____

_____

_____

Mood
How do you feel right now?
(Circle the one that represents how you feel.)

Energy Level
(Just notice— this isn't about motivation.)

How do I want to feel today?
(Write a word or phrase, or circle one.)

CALM • LIGHTER • STEADY • CONFIDENT
SAFE • FOCUSED • MYSELF

_____

_____

Today's Affirmation or Intention
(Keep it simple. One sentence is enough.)

_____

_____

Today, I give myself permission to take this one step at a time.

Evening Reflection

You made it through the day. That matters.

Mood
How did you feel overall today?

What challenged me today?
(Externally or internally—both count.)

_____

_____

_____

What helped me feel even a little stronger or lighter today? (Small things matter more than you think.)

_____

_____

_____

One thing I'm grateful for today:
(It can be about yourself, someone else, or a quiet moment.)

_____

_____

_____

Gentle Reminder: *If today felt heavy, that doesn't mean you failed. It means you showed up—and that's enough for today.*

TODAY'S LETTING-GO PRACTICE: Identify the Burden

The burden this week is your resistance to joy. What is one thought that blocks you from feeling good or having fun? (E.g., "I don't have time," "I don't deserve it," "It's not productive.")

_____

_____

_____

_____

_____

_____

_____

DAY 72

Morning Intention

Take a breath before you begin.

What am I noticing in myself this morning? (Thoughts, emotions, body sensations—anything that stands out.)

_____

_____

_____

Mood
How do you feel right now?
(Circle the one that represents how you feel.)

Energy Level
(Just notice— this isn't about motivation.)

How do I want to feel today?
(Write a word or phrase, or circle one.)

CALM • LIGHTER • STEADY • CONFIDENT
SAFE • FOCUSED • MYSELF

_____

_____

Today's Affirmation or Intention
(Keep it simple. One sentence is enough.)

_____

_____

_____

Today, I give myself permission to take this one step at a time.

Evening Reflection

You made it through the day. That matters.

Mood
How did you feel overall today?

What challenged me today?
(Externally or internally—both count.)

_____

_____

_____

What helped me feel even a little stronger or lighter today? (Small things matter more than you think.)

_____

_____

_____

One thing I'm grateful for today:
(It can be about yourself, someone else, or a quiet moment.)

_____

_____

_____

Gentle Reminder: *If today felt heavy, that doesn't mean you failed. It means you showed up—and that's enough for today.*

TODAY'S LETTING-GO PRACTICE: Write to Understand

Today's practice is a joy list exercise. Brainstorm and write down
10 activities, big or small, that bring you a feeling of pure joy. Don't
overthink it; just list what comes to mind.

_____

_____

_____

_____

_____

_____

_____

_____

DAY 73

Morning Intention

Take a breath before you begin.

What am I noticing in myself this morning? (Thoughts, emotions, body sensations—anything that stands out.)

_____

_____

_____

Mood
How do you feel right now?
(Circle the one that represents how you feel.)

Energy Level
(Just notice—this isn't about motivation.)

How do I want to feel today?
(Write a word or phrase, or circle one.)

CALM • LIGHTER • STEADY • CONFIDENT
SAFE • FOCUSED • MYSELF

_____

_____

Today's Affirmation or Intention
(Keep it simple. One sentence is enough.)

_____

_____

_____

Today, I give myself permission to take this one step at a time.

Evening Reflection

You made it through the day. That matters.

Mood
How did you feel overall today?

What challenged me today?
(Externally or internally—both count.)

_____

_____

_____

What helped me feel even a little stronger or lighter today? (Small things matter more than you think.)

_____

_____

_____

One thing I'm grateful for today:
(It can be about yourself, someone else, or a quiet moment.)

_____

_____

_____

Gentle Reminder: *If today felt heavy, that doesn't mean you failed. It means you showed up—and that's enough for today.*

TODAY'S LETTING-GO PRACTICE: Act of Release

Choose one activity from your joy list and do it today. The goal is to do one thing purely for fun, without guilt. Release the need for everything to be productive.

DAY 74

Morning Intention	Evening Reflection

Morning Intention

Take a breath before you begin.

What am I noticing in myself this morning? (Thoughts, emotions, body sensations—anything that stands out.)

_____

_____

_____

Mood
How do you feel right now?
(Circle the one that represents how you feel.)

Energy Level
(Just notice—
this isn't about
motivation.)

How do I want to feel today?
(Write a word or phrase, or circle one.)

CALM • LIGHTER • STEADY • CONFIDENT
SAFE • FOCUSED • MYSELF

_____

_____

Today's Affirmation or Intention
(Keep it simple. One sentence is enough.)

_____

_____

_____

*Today, I give myself permission
to take this one step at a time.*

Evening Reflection

*You made it through the day.
That matters.*

Mood
How did you feel overall today?

What challenged me today?
(Externally or internally—both count.)

_____

_____

_____

What helped me feel even a little stronger or lighter today? (Small things matter more than you think.)

_____

_____

_____

One thing I'm grateful for today:
(It can be about yourself, someone else, or a quiet moment.)

_____

_____

_____

Gentle Reminder: *If today felt heavy, that doesn't mean you failed. It means you showed up—and that's enough for today.*

TODAY'S LETTING-GO PRACTICE: Mindful Detachment

While you are doing (or thinking about) a joyful activity, you might notice thoughts of guilt. Practice noticing these thoughts without latching onto them. Label them "joy blockers" and let them float by, then return your focus to the pleasant feeling.

_____

_____

_____

_____

_____

_____

_____

DAY 75

Morning Intention

Take a breath before you begin.

What am I noticing in myself this morning? (Thoughts, emotions, body sensations—anything that stands out.)

_____

_____

_____

Mood
How do you feel right now?
(Circle the one that represents how you feel.)

Energy Level
(Just notice— this isn't about motivation.)

How do I want to feel today?
(Write a word or phrase, or circle one.)

CALM • LIGHTER • STEADY • CONFIDENT
SAFE • FOCUSED • MYSELF

_____

_____

Today's Affirmation or Intention
(Keep it simple. One sentence is enough.)

_____

_____

_____

Today, I give myself permission to take this one step at a time.

Evening Reflection

You made it through the day. That matters.

Mood
How did you feel overall today?

What challenged me today?
(Externally or internally—both count.)

_____

_____

_____

What helped me feel even a little stronger or lighter today? (Small things matter more than you think.)

_____

_____

_____

One thing I'm grateful for today:
(It can be about yourself, someone else, or a quiet moment.)

_____

_____

_____

Gentle Reminder: *If today felt heavy, that doesn't mean you failed. It means you showed up—and that's enough for today.*

TODAY'S LETTING-GO PRACTICE:
Reclaim Your Peace (Boundaries)

Your boundary today is against feelings of unworthiness. When the thought "I don't deserve it" comes up, replace it with, "I am open to receiving."

DAY 76

Morning Intention

Take a breath before you begin.

What am I noticing in myself this morning? (Thoughts, emotions, body sensations—anything that stands out.)

_____

_____

_____

Mood
How do you feel right now?
(Circle the one that represents how you feel.)

Energy Level
(Just notice—this isn't about motivation.)

How do I want to feel today?
(Write a word or phrase, or circle one.)

CALM • LIGHTER • STEADY • CONFIDENT
SAFE • FOCUSED • MYSELF

_____

_____

Today's Affirmation or Intention
(Keep it simple. One sentence is enough.)

_____

_____

_____

Today, I give myself permission to take this one step at a time.

Evening Reflection

You made it through the day. That matters.

Mood
How did you feel overall today?

What challenged me today?
(Externally or internally—both count.)

_____

_____

_____

What helped me feel even a little stronger or lighter today? (Small things matter more than you think.)

_____

_____

_____

One thing I'm grateful for today:
(It can be about yourself, someone else, or a quiet moment.)

_____

_____

_____

Gentle Reminder: *If today felt heavy, that doesn't mean you failed. It means you showed up—and that's enough for today.*

TODAY'S LETTING-GO PRACTICE: Express and Externalize

Find one song that reliably makes you feel joyful. Put it on and just listen. Let the music be the focus. Notice how it feels in your body. This is an act of intentionally inviting joy into your space.

DAY 77

Morning Intention

Take a breath before you begin.

What am I noticing in myself this morning? (Thoughts, emotions, body sensations—anything that stands out.)

_____

_____

_____

Mood
How do you feel right now?
(Circle the one that represents how you feel.)

Energy Level
(Just notice—this isn't about motivation.)

How do I want to feel today?
(Write a word or phrase, or circle one.)

CALM • LIGHTER • STEADY • CONFIDENT
SAFE • FOCUSED • MYSELF

_____

_____

Today's Affirmation or Intention
(Keep it simple. One sentence is enough.)

_____

_____

_____

Today, I give myself permission to take this one step at a time.

Evening Reflection

You made it through the day. That matters.

Mood
How did you feel overall today?

What challenged me today?
(Externally or internally—both count.)

_____

_____

_____

What helped me feel even a little stronger or lighter today? (Small things matter more than you think.)

_____

_____

_____

One thing I'm grateful for today:
(It can be about yourself, someone else, or a quiet moment.)

_____

_____

_____

Gentle Reminder: *If today felt heavy, that doesn't mean you failed. It means you showed up—and that's enough for today.*

TODAY'S LETTING-GO PRACTICE: Notice the Lightness

This is your End-of-Week Reflection. How did you embrace joy this week? How did it feel to intentionally make space for it?

_____

_____

_____

_____

_____

_____

_____

YOGA POSE: Reclining Butterfly

Gently opens hips/groin, calms mind, and relieves stress/mild depression, creating a sense of openness and receptivity to joy.

BREATHWORK EXERCISE: Sighing Breath

Releases stress and promotes immediate relaxation, helping to let go of any resistance to experiencing pure joy.

See appendix at the back of the book for more details
on Yoga Poses and Breathwork Exercises.

I am the architect
of my peace.

Sustaining Your Strength

DAY 78

Morning Intention

Take a breath before you begin.

What am I noticing in myself this morning? (Thoughts, emotions, body sensations—anything that stands out.)

_____

_____

_____

Mood
How do you feel right now?
(Circle the one that represents how you feel.)

Energy Level
(Just notice—this isn't about motivation.)

How do I want to feel today?
(Write a word or phrase, or circle one.)

CALM • LIGHTER • STEADY • CONFIDENT
SAFE • FOCUSED • MYSELF

_____

_____

Today's Affirmation or Intention
(Keep it simple. One sentence is enough.)

_____

_____

_____

Today, I give myself permission to take this one step at a time.

Evening Reflection

*You made it through the day.
That matters.*

Mood
How did you feel overall today?

What challenged me today?
(Externally or internally—both count.)

_____

_____

_____

What helped me feel even a little stronger or lighter today? (Small things matter more than you think.)

_____

_____

_____

One thing I'm grateful for today:
(It can be about yourself, someone else, or a quiet moment.)

_____

_____

_____

Gentle Reminder: *If today felt heavy, that doesn't mean you failed. It means you showed up—and that's enough for today.*

TODAY'S LETTING-GO PRACTICE: Identify the Burden

The final burden is the fear of losing your progress. What is your biggest fear or doubt about sustaining your strength after this journey ends (e.g., the fear that you'll fall back into old, unhealthy habits)?

_____

_____

_____

_____

_____

_____

_____

DAY 79

Morning Intention

Take a breath before you begin.

What am I noticing in myself this morning? (Thoughts, emotions, body sensations—anything that stands out.)

_____

_____

_____

Mood
How do you feel right now?
(Circle the one that represents how you feel.)

Energy Level
(Just notice— this isn't about motivation.)

How do I want to feel today?
(Write a word or phrase, or circle one.)

CALM • LIGHTER • STEADY • CONFIDENT
SAFE • FOCUSED • MYSELF

_____

_____

Today's Affirmation or Intention
(Keep it simple. One sentence is enough.)

_____

_____

_____

Today, I give myself permission to take this one step at a time.

Evening Reflection

You made it through the day. That matters.

Mood
How did you feel overall today?

What challenged me today?
(Externally or internally—both count.)

_____

_____

_____

What helped me feel even a little stronger or lighter today? (Small things matter more than you think.)

_____

_____

_____

One thing I'm grateful for today:
(It can be about yourself, someone else, or a quiet moment.)

_____

_____

_____

Gentle Reminder: *If today felt heavy, that doesn't mean you failed. It means you showed up—and that's enough for today.*

TODAY'S LETTING-GO PRACTICE: Write to Understand

Today, you will write a letter to your future self. Write a letter to yourself six months from now, celebrating the 90-day journey you've just completed. Remind your future self of the tools you've learned and the strength you've built.

_____

_____

_____

_____

_____

_____

_____

DAY 80

Morning Intention

Take a breath before you begin.

What am I noticing in myself this morning? (Thoughts, emotions, body sensations—anything that stands out.)

_____

_____

_____

Mood
How do you feel right now?
(Circle the one that represents how you feel.)

Energy Level
(Just notice—
this isn't about
motivation.)

How do I want to feel today?
(Write a word or phrase, or circle one.)

CALM • LIGHTER • STEADY • CONFIDENT
SAFE • FOCUSED • MYSELF

_____

_____

Today's Affirmation or Intention
(Keep it simple. One sentence is enough.)

_____

_____

_____

*Today, I give myself permission
to take this one step at a time.*

Evening Reflection

*You made it through the day.
That matters.*

Mood
How did you feel overall today?

What challenged me today?
(Externally or internally—both count.)

_____

_____

_____

What helped me feel even a little stronger or lighter today? (Small things matter more than you think.)

_____

_____

_____

One thing I'm grateful for today:
(It can be about yourself, someone else, or a quiet moment.)

_____

_____

_____

Gentle Reminder: *If today felt heavy, that doesn't mean you failed. It means you showed up—and that's enough for today.*

TODAY'S LETTING-GO PRACTICE: Act of Release

Your action today is to commit to your future peace. Plan one new self-care habit to continue. Write down the habit and the first small, concrete step you will take to implement it.

_____

_____

_____

_____

_____

_____

_____

_____

DAY 81

Morning Intention

Take a breath before you begin.

What am I noticing in myself this morning? (Thoughts, emotions, body sensations—anything that stands out.)

_____

_____

_____

Mood
How do you feel right now?
(Circle the one that represents how you feel.)

Energy Level
(Just notice—this isn't about motivation.)

How do I want to feel today?
(Write a word or phrase, or circle one.)

CALM • LIGHTER • STEADY • CONFIDENT
SAFE • FOCUSED • MYSELF

_____

_____

Today's Affirmation or Intention
(Keep it simple. One sentence is enough.)

_____

_____

_____

Today, I give myself permission to take this one step at a time.

Evening Reflection

You made it through the day. That matters.

Mood
How did you feel overall today?

What challenged me today?
(Externally or internally—both count.)

_____

_____

_____

What helped me feel even a little stronger or lighter today? (Small things matter more than you think.)

_____

_____

_____

One thing I'm grateful for today:
(It can be about yourself, someone else, or a quiet moment.)

_____

_____

_____

Gentle Reminder: *If today felt heavy, that doesn't mean you failed. It means you showed up—and that's enough for today.*

TODAY'S LETTING-GO PRACTICE: Mindful Detachment

Healing is not a straight line; it is a spiral. If you have a moment of setback, you might think, "I've failed." Practice noticing this all-or-nothing thought. Label it "thinking" and remind yourself that revisiting old feelings is natural, and you are not starting from scratch.

_____

_____

_____

_____

_____

_____

_____

DAY 82

Morning Intention

Take a breath before you begin.

What am I noticing in myself this morning? (Thoughts, emotions, body sensations—anything that stands out.)

_____

_____

_____

Mood
How do you feel right now?
(Circle the one that represents how you feel.)

Energy Level
(Just notice—this isn't about motivation.)

How do I want to feel today?
(Write a word or phrase, or circle one.)

CALM • LIGHTER • STEADY • CONFIDENT
SAFE • FOCUSED • MYSELF

_____

_____

Today's Affirmation or Intention
(Keep it simple. One sentence is enough.)

_____

_____

_____

Today, I give myself permission to take this one step at a time.

Evening Reflection

You made it through the day. That matters.

Mood
How did you feel overall today?

What challenged me today?
(Externally or internally—both count.)

_____

_____

_____

What helped me feel even a little stronger or lighter today? (Small things matter more than you think.)

_____

_____

_____

One thing I'm grateful for today:
(It can be about yourself, someone else, or a quiet moment.)

_____

_____

Gentle Reminder: *If today felt heavy, that doesn't mean you failed. It means you showed up—and that's enough for today.*

TODAY'S LETTING-GO PRACTICE:
Reclaim Your Peace (Boundaries)

Your boundary is against the fear of regression. When the thought "I'll fall back into old, unhealthy habits" arises, firmly replace it with the affirmation "I'm building new patterns."

DAY 83

Morning Intention

Take a breath before you begin.

What am I noticing in myself this morning? (Thoughts, emotions, body sensations—anything that stands out.)

_____

_____

_____

Mood
How do you feel right now?
(Circle the one that represents how you feel.)

Energy Level
(Just notice—
this isn't about
motivation.)

How do I want to feel today?
(Write a word or phrase, or circle one.)

CALM • LIGHTER • STEADY • CONFIDENT
SAFE • FOCUSED • MYSELF

_____

_____

Today's Affirmation or Intention
(Keep it simple. One sentence is enough.)

_____

_____

_____

*Today, I give myself permission
to take this one step at a time.*

Evening Reflection

*You made it through the day.
That matters.*

Mood
How did you feel overall today?

What challenged me today?
(Externally or internally—both count.)

_____

_____

_____

What helped me feel even a little stronger or lighter today? (Small things matter more than you think.)

_____

_____

_____

One thing I'm grateful for today:
(It can be about yourself, someone else, or a quiet moment.)

_____

_____

_____

Gentle Reminder: *If today felt heavy, that doesn't mean you failed. It means you showed up—and that's enough for today.*

TODAY'S LETTING-GO PRACTICE: Express and Externalize

Look back through the past 11 weeks of this journal. Find the one mantra, prompt, or insight that was most meaningful to you. Write it below or on a separate piece of paper and decorate it. This is your personal touchstone to carry forward.

_____

_____

_____

_____

_____

_____

_____

DAY 84

Morning Intention

Take a breath before you begin.

What am I noticing in myself this morning? (Thoughts, emotions, body sensations—anything that stands out.)

_____

_____

_____

Mood
How do you feel right now?
(Circle the one that represents how you feel.)

Energy Level
(Just notice—this isn't about motivation.)

How do I want to feel today?
(Write a word or phrase, or circle one.)

CALM • LIGHTER • STEADY • CONFIDENT
SAFE • FOCUSED • MYSELF

_____

_____

Today's Affirmation or Intention
(Keep it simple. One sentence is enough.)

_____

_____

_____

Today, I give myself permission to take this one step at a time.

Evening Reflection

You made it through the day. That matters.

Mood
How did you feel overall today?

What challenged me today?
(Externally or internally—both count.)

_____

_____

_____

What helped me feel even a little stronger or lighter today? (Small things matter more than you think.)

_____

_____

_____

One thing I'm grateful for today:
(It can be about yourself, someone else, or a quiet moment.)

_____

_____

_____

Gentle Reminder: *If today felt heavy, that doesn't mean you failed. It means you showed up—and that's enough for today.*

TODAY'S LETTING-GO PRACTICE: Notice the Lightness

This is your End-of-Week Reflection. The mantra is "I am the architect of my peace." Reflect on Day 80's question: What new self-care habit will I carry forward? Write down your commitment to yourself and your ongoing journey.

_____

_____

_____

_____

_____

_____

_____

_____

YOGA POSE: Bridge Pose

Strengthens back/glutes/hamstrings, opens chest, and calms brain, reinforcing physical and mental strength for continued well-being.

BREATHWORK EXERCISE: Humming Bee Breath

Calms nerves, reduces stress/anxiety, and improves focus, supporting a sustained sense of inner peace and resilience.

See appendix at the back of the book for more details
on Yoga Poses and Breathwork Exercises.

REFLECTION ON THE PAST 4 WEEKS

What was your biggest insight or breakthrough during the last four weeks?

_____

_____

_____

_____

_____

_____

_____

What challenge did you face, and how did you overcome it (or what did you learn from it)?

_____

_____

_____

_____

_____

_____

_____

REFLECTION ON THE PAST 4 WEEKS

What is one thing you are grateful for from these past four weeks?

_____

_____

_____

_____

_____

_____

_____

_____

How has your sense of peace or understanding of "letting go" evolved?

_____

_____

_____

_____

_____

_____

_____

_____

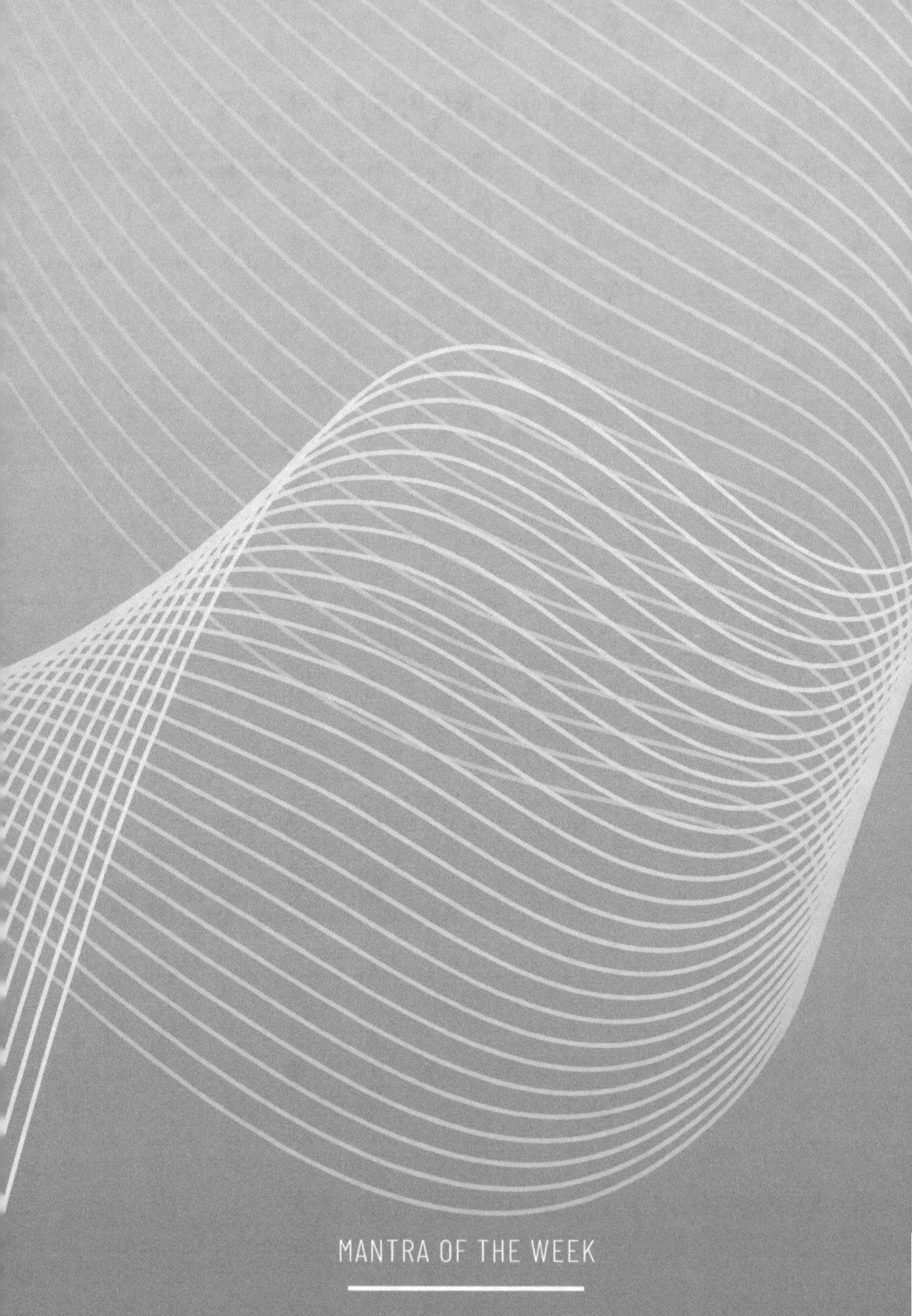

MANTRA OF THE WEEK

I am the architect of my life.

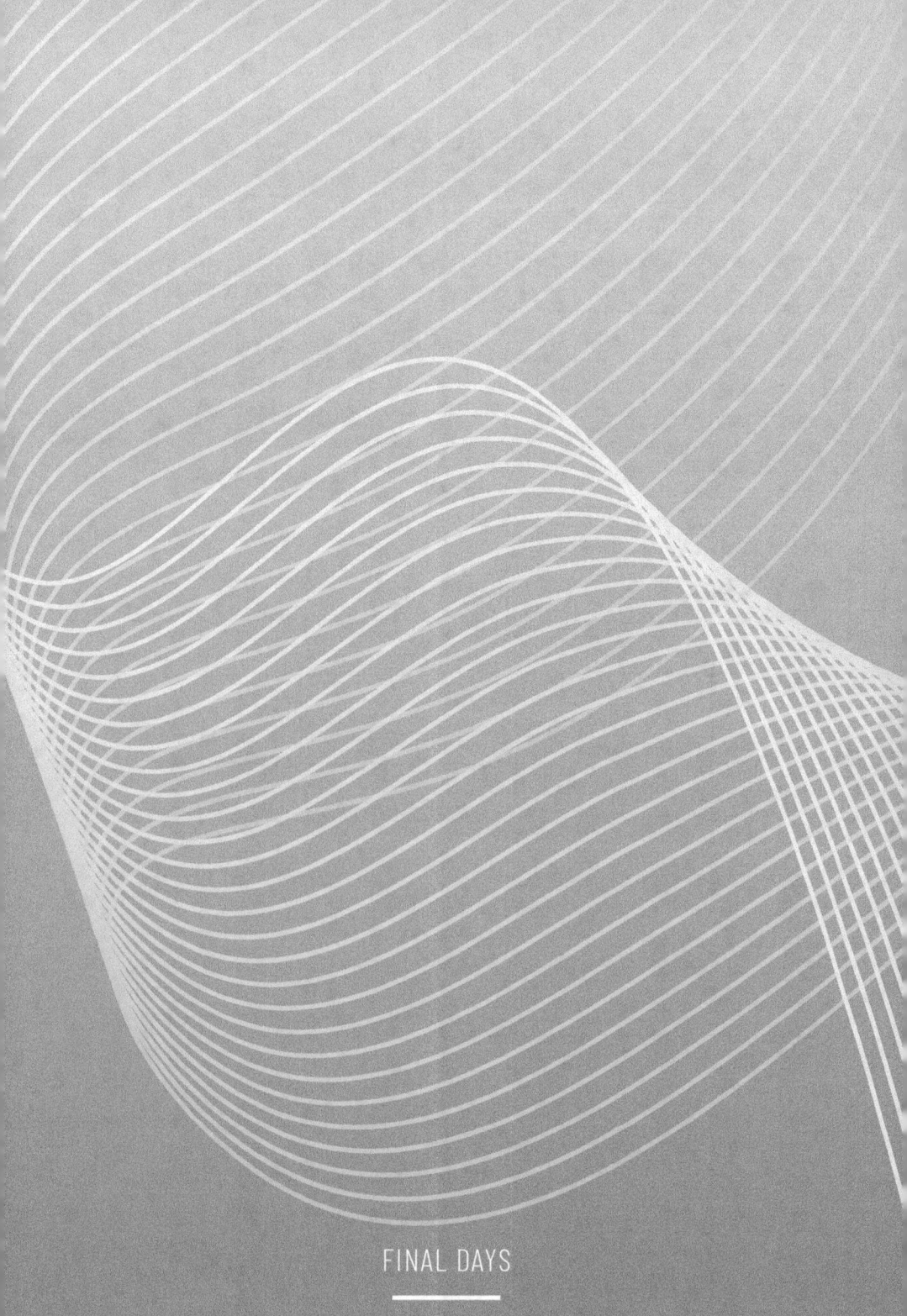

FINAL DAYS

Integration and Moving Forward

DAY 85

Morning Intention

Take a breath before you begin.

What am I noticing in myself this morning? (Thoughts, emotions, body sensations—anything that stands out.)

_____

_____

_____

Mood
How do you feel right now?
(Circle the one that represents how you feel.)

Energy Level
(Just notice—
this isn't about
motivation.)

How do I want to feel today?
(Write a word or phrase, or circle one.)

CALM • LIGHTER • STEADY • CONFIDENT
SAFE • FOCUSED • MYSELF

_____

_____

Today's Affirmation or Intention
(Keep it simple. One sentence is enough.)

_____

_____

_____

*Today, I give myself permission
to take this one step at a time.*

Evening Reflection

*You made it through the day.
That matters.*

Mood
How did you feel overall today?

What challenged me today?
(Externally or internally—both count.)

_____

_____

_____

What helped me feel even a little stronger or lighter today? (Small things matter more than you think.)

_____

_____

_____

One thing I'm grateful for today:
(It can be about yourself, someone else, or a quiet moment.)

_____

_____

_____

Gentle Reminder: *If today felt heavy, that doesn't mean you failed. It means you showed up—and that's enough for today.*

TODAY'S LETTING-GO PRACTICE: Revisit Facing the Pain

Think back to the pain you identified in Week 1. How has your relationship with that pain changed, even slightly, over the past three months?

_____

_____

_____

_____

_____

_____

_____

DAY 86

Morning Intention

Take a breath before you begin.

What am I noticing in myself this morning? (Thoughts, emotions, body sensations—anything that stands out.)

_____

_____

_____

Mood
How do you feel right now?
(Circle the one that represents how you feel.)

Energy Level
(Just notice—this isn't about motivation.)

How do I want to feel today?
(Write a word or phrase, or circle one.)

CALM • LIGHTER • STEADY • CONFIDENT
SAFE • FOCUSED • MYSELF

_____

_____

Today's Affirmation or Intention
(Keep it simple. One sentence is enough.)

_____

_____

_____

Today, I give myself permission to take this one step at a time.

Evening Reflection

You made it through the day. That matters.

Mood
How did you feel overall today?

What challenged me today?
(Externally or internally—both count.)

_____

_____

_____

What helped me feel even a little stronger or lighter today? (Small things matter more than you think.)

_____

_____

_____

One thing I'm grateful for today:
(It can be about yourself, someone else, or a quiet moment.)

_____

_____

Gentle Reminder: *If today felt heavy, that doesn't mean you failed. It means you showed up—and that's enough for today.*

TODAY'S LETTING-GO PRACTICE: Revisit Boundaries

Think about the boundaries you practiced in Week 8. What is one boundary that has been most important in protecting your peace?

_____

_____

_____

_____

_____

_____

_____

DAY 87

Morning Intention

Take a breath before you begin.

What am I noticing in myself this morning? (Thoughts, emotions, body sensations—anything that stands out.)

_____

_____

_____

Mood
How do you feel right now?
(Circle the one that represents how you feel.)

Energy Level
(Just notice—this isn't about motivation.)

How do I want to feel today?
(Write a word or phrase, or circle one.)

CALM • LIGHTER • STEADY • CONFIDENT
SAFE • FOCUSED • MYSELF

_____

_____

Today's Affirmation or Intention
(Keep it simple. One sentence is enough.)

_____

_____

_____

Today, I give myself permission to take this one step at a time.

Evening Reflection

You made it through the day. That matters.

Mood
How did you feel overall today?

What challenged me today?
(Externally or internally—both count.)

_____

_____

_____

What helped me feel even a little stronger or lighter today? (Small things matter more than you think.)

_____

_____

_____

One thing I'm grateful for today:
(It can be about yourself, someone else, or a quiet moment.)

_____

_____

_____

Gentle Reminder: *If today felt heavy, that doesn't mean you failed. It means you showed up—and that's enough for today.*

TODAY'S LETTING-GO PRACTICE: Revisit Self-Forgiveness

Consider the mantra from Week 6: "I deserve my own compassion."
What does an act of self-compassion look like for you today?

_____

_____

_____

_____

_____

_____

_____

DAY 88

Morning Intention

Take a breath before you begin.

What am I noticing in myself this morning? (Thoughts, emotions, body sensations—anything that stands out.)

_____

_____

_____

Mood
How do you feel right now?
(Circle the one that represents how you feel.)

Energy Level
(Just notice—this isn't about motivation.)

How do I want to feel today?
(Write a word or phrase, or circle one.)

CALM • LIGHTER • STEADY • CONFIDENT
SAFE • FOCUSED • MYSELF

_____

_____

Today's Affirmation or Intention
(Keep it simple. One sentence is enough.)

_____

_____

_____

Today, I give myself permission to take this one step at a time.

Evening Reflection

You made it through the day. That matters.

Mood
How did you feel overall today?

What challenged me today?
(Externally or internally—both count.)

_____

_____

_____

What helped me feel even a little stronger or lighter today? (Small things matter more than you think.)

_____

_____

_____

One thing I'm grateful for today:
(It can be about yourself, someone else, or a quiet moment.)

_____

_____

_____

Gentle Reminder: *If today felt heavy, that doesn't mean you failed. It means you showed up—and that's enough for today.*

TODAY'S LETTING-GO PRACTICE: Revisit Gratitude

Look back on this entire journey. Name three things you are grateful for about your own strength and resilience.

_____

_____

_____

_____

_____

_____

_____

DAY 89

Morning Intention

Take a breath before you begin.

What am I noticing in myself this morning? (Thoughts, emotions, body sensations—anything that stands out.)

_____

_____

_____

Mood
How do you feel right now?
(Circle the one that represents how you feel.)

Energy Level
(Just notice—this isn't about motivation.)

How do I want to feel today?
(Write a word or phrase, or circle one.)

CALM • LIGHTER • STEADY • CONFIDENT
SAFE • FOCUSED • MYSELF

_____

_____

Today's Affirmation or Intention
(Keep it simple. One sentence is enough.)

_____

_____

_____

Today, I give myself permission to take this one step at a time.

Evening Reflection

You made it through the day. That matters.

Mood
How did you feel overall today?

What challenged me today?
(Externally or internally—both count.)

_____

_____

_____

What helped me feel even a little stronger or lighter today? (Small things matter more than you think.)

_____

_____

_____

One thing I'm grateful for today:
(It can be about yourself, someone else, or a quiet moment.)

_____

_____

_____

Gentle Reminder: *If today felt heavy, that doesn't mean you failed. It means you showed up—and that's enough for today.*

TODAY'S LETTING-GO PRACTICE: Revisit Joy

Think about your joy list from Week 11. What is one small joy you can intentionally create for yourself in the next 24 hours?

_____

_____

_____

_____

_____

_____

_____

_____

DAY 90

Morning Intention

Take a breath before you begin.

What am I noticing in myself this morning? (Thoughts, emotions, body sensations—anything that stands out.)

_____

_____

_____

Mood
How do you feel right now?
(Circle the one that represents how you feel.)

Energy Level
(Just notice—
this isn't about
motivation.)

How do I want to feel today?
(Write a word or phrase, or circle one.)

CALM • LIGHTER • STEADY • CONFIDENT
SAFE • FOCUSED • MYSELF

_____

_____

Today's Affirmation or Intention
(Keep it simple. One sentence is enough.)

_____

_____

_____

*Today, I give myself permission
to take this one step at a time.*

Evening Reflection

*You made it through the day.
That matters.*

Mood
How did you feel overall today?

What challenged me today?
(Externally or internally—both count.)

_____

_____

_____

What helped me feel even a little stronger or lighter today? (Small things matter more than you think.)

_____

_____

_____

One thing I'm grateful for today:
(It can be about yourself, someone else, or a quiet moment.)

_____

_____

_____

Gentle Reminder: *If today felt heavy, that doesn't mean you failed. It means you showed up—and that's enough for today.*

TODAY'S LETTING-GO PRACTICE: A Final Intention

Based on everything you have learned and practiced, write one final intention for the next chapter of your life. What will you carry forward?

_____

_____

_____

_____

_____

_____

_____

YOGA POSE: Easy Pose

A gentle, grounding pose for reflection and integration, symbolizing peace and continued practice.

BREATHWORK EXERCISE: Resonant Breathing

Helps maintain balance and a sense of calm as you integrate your journey and move forward with newfound strength.

See appendix at the back of the book for more details
on Yoga Poses and Breathwork Exercises.

As You Move Forward
A Self-Assessment

You've come so far on your healing journey. Take a moment to honestly reflect on where you are right now. This is not a test; it's a snapshot of your current emotional landscape.

Note: To complete this self-assessment, use the rating scale provided in the instructions below to evaluate each statement.

INSTRUCTIONS

Rate yourself on a scale of 1 to 5, where:

> 1 = Strongly Disagree
> 2 = Disagree
> 3 = Neutral
> 4 = Agree
> 5 = Strongly Agree

EMOTIONAL WELL-BEING SELF-ASSESSMENT

1. I feel strong enough to face difficult emotions.

2. I can identify situations or thoughts that trigger my pain.

3. I feel comfortable expressing my true feelings and needs.

4. I am able to forgive myself for past mistakes or perceived shortcomings.

5. I feel a sense of worthiness and self-acceptance.

6. I have clear boundaries that protect my energy.

7. I regularly experience feelings of gratitude.

8. I feel hopeful about my future and can envision positive change.

9. I allow myself to experience joy without guilt.

10. I feel equipped to handle setbacks and maintain my peace.

REFLECT ON YOUR SCORES

Which areas did you rate lowest? These might be key areas to focus on as you move forward.

Which areas did you rate highest? Acknowledge your existing strengths!

Compare your results to the self-assessment you completed before beginning this journey. Where have you improved? Celebrate your progress!

What is one feeling you are most proud to have cultivated by completing this journal?

A Final Note of Encouragement

Congratulations on completing this 90-day journey. The commitment you made to yourself is a profound act of love and courage. Remember that healing is not a linear path with a final destination. It is a spiral, and there will be days you feel like you are soaring and other days you may revisit old feelings. This is normal and natural.

The difference is that you are no longer starting from scratch. You now possess a toolkit of practices—gratitude, mindfulness, self-compassion, boundary-setting—that you can return to whenever you need. You have proven to yourself that you have the strength to face your burdens, the wisdom to learn from them, and the resilience to rise.

Continue to be gentle with yourself. Keep choosing progress over perfection. Your journey is uniquely yours, and you have everything you need within you to navigate it with grace.

Certificate of Freedom

This certifies that

Name: _____

has successfully completed the 90-day guided journal
for letting go, marking a powerful first step toward
choosing freedom, resilience, and self-respect.

Date: _____

Appendix

BREATHE, RELEASE, RESTORE

7 Days to Emotional Healing and Inner Peace

You get a FREE 7-day guided video experience built to help you calm your mind, reset your energy, and feel lighter every day. In this video course, you'll find:

- Instructions for the seven breathing strategies shared in the journal
- Step-by-step guidance to practice eight empowering yoga poses
- Opportunities for reflection and self-assessment to complement your journey through this journal

You can use these complementary videos as guidance as you work through each week's breathing and yoga exercises. The following pages of the appendix also break down the yoga poses and breathwork exercises you'll use throughout your journey.

Scan the QR code below or visit
www.BreatheReleaseRestore.com
to begin your 7-day reset.

BREATHE. RELEASE. RESTORE.

YOGA POSES

Integrating yoga into your daily routine is an effective method for alleviating stress, soothing your thoughts, and enhancing your overall health. These straightforward yoga poses are designed to engage both your body and mind, facilitating the release of tension and the attainment of equilibrium. Practicing these poses can significantly reduce your stress levels and promote relaxation.

Standing Forward Bend

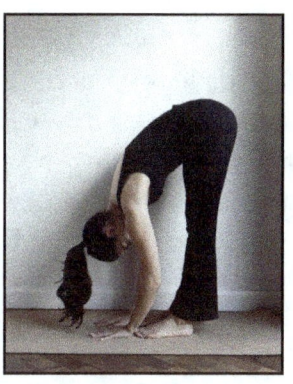

HOW TO PRACTICE

1. Stand tall with feet hip-width apart.
2. Exhale and slowly bend forward, keeping a slight bend in your knees.
3. Place your palms on the floor, letting your head rest against your legs.
4. Stretch your spine in different directions as you pull your head down.
5. For a deeper stretch, straighten your legs.
6. Hold for six to eight breaths.
7. Inhale, slowly raise your arms and torso back to standing.

The Standing Forward Bend promotes flexibility and relaxation. Following these steps helps release tension in your legs and back, allowing relaxation to envelop each part of your body.

Cat-Cow Pose

HOW TO PRACTICE

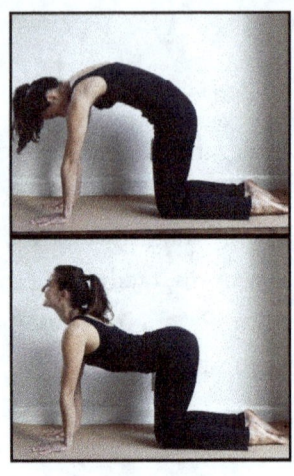

1. Start on all fours, with wrists directly under your shoulders and knees under your hips.
2. Inhale and hold your breath.
3. **Cat:** Exhale and round your back toward the ceiling, bringing your navel toward your spine.
4. Return to the neutral position with a straight back.
5. **Cow:** Inhale, tilt your pelvis back, and lift your tailbone up while drawing your navel in and keeping your spine aligned.
6. Continue to flow between Cat and Cow for several breaths.

Incorporating Cat-Cow Pose into your routine promotes spinal flexibility and relieves tension. This gentle flow enhances body awareness, making it an ideal exercise for relaxation and mindfulness.

Easy Pose

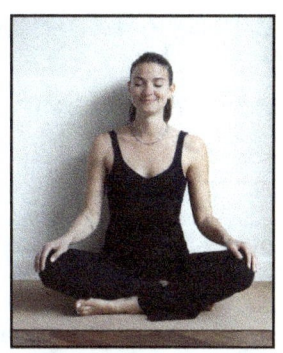

HOW TO PRACTICE

1. Sit on the floor with your legs extended in front of you.
2. Cross your legs, placing each foot beneath the opposite knee.
3. Rest your palms on your knees, with your fingers pointing down.
4. Align your head, neck, and spine, sitting upright with balanced weight.
5. Lengthen your spine while softening your neck, and gently relax your feet and thighs.
6. Stay for about a minute, then switch the cross of your legs.

Practicing Easy Pose fosters relaxation and mindfulness, enhancing your overall well-being. Regularly incorporating this pose into your routine can improve flexibility and aid in achieving mental clarity.

Bridge Pose

HOW TO PRACTICE

1. Lie on your back with knees bent and feet flat on the floor, hip-width apart.
2. Place your arms at your sides with palms facing down.
3. Inhale and lift your hips off the floor, rolling your spine up.
4. Squeeze your knees together to keep them aligned, and press your arms and shoulders into the floor to lift your chest.
5. Engage your legs and glutes to raise your hips higher.
6. Hold the pose for four to eight breaths, then slowly lower your hips back to the floor.

Bridge Pose is an excellent way to strengthen the back, glutes, and legs while promoting flexibility in the spine. Regular practice can enhance posture and relieve stress-related tension in the body.

Downward-Facing Dog

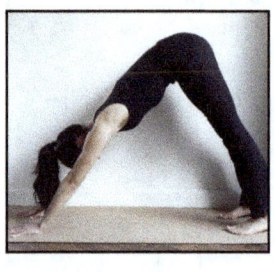

HOW TO PRACTICE

1. Start in a tabletop position.
2. Lift your hips up and back, forming an inverted V shape.
3. Keep your hands shoulder-width apart and press your heels toward the ground.
4. Hold for 5–10 breaths.

Reclining Butterfly

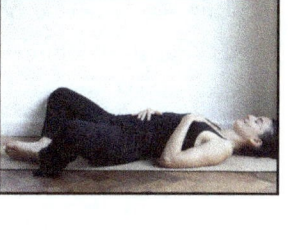

HOW TO PRACTICE

1. Lie on your back and bring the soles of your feet together.
2. Let your knees fall open like butterfly wings.
3. Place one hand on your heart and one on your belly, breathing deeply.

Supine Twist

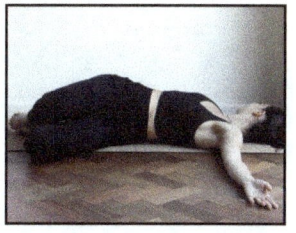

HOW TO PRACTICE

1. Lie on your back and bring one knee to your chest.
2. Gently twist the knee across your body while keeping your shoulders on the floor.
3. Extend your opposite arm and gaze in the opposite direction.
4. Hold for a few breaths, then switch sides.

Legs Up the Wall

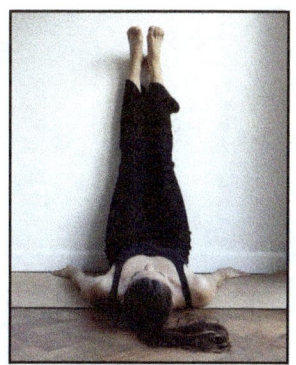

HOW TO PRACTICE

1. Sit sideways against a wall.
2. Swing your legs up and rest them against the wall.
3. Lie back with arms relaxed by your sides and breathe deeply.

Regular practice of these yoga poses leads to a reduction in stress and anxiety while enhancing both mental and physical health. Moving at your own pace and focusing on your breath is essential, as each pose helps to reconnect with your body and release any tension. With consistent practice, these simple yet effective poses become a vital part of your self-care routine, promoting peace and relaxation in your daily life.

BREATHWORK EXERCISES

Breathing is an often-overlooked yet powerful tool in stress management. By tapping into various breathing techniques, you can create a sense of calm and presence, easing stress and anxiety. In this section, we explore several effective breathing practices designed to help you ground yourself in the present moment and help manage stress. These exercises can be performed in various locations; however, it is recommended that you practice these techniques in tranquil, open spaces with minimal auditory distractions.

Deep Diaphragmatic Breathing

Unlike shallow chest breathing, deep diaphragmatic breathing engages the diaphragm, allowing the lungs to fill completely and promoting relaxation. This technique lowers your heart rate, reduces tension, and helps you feel more grounded.

HOW TO PRACTICE

1. Sit comfortably and place one hand on your abdomen.
2. Inhale deeply through your nose, letting your abdomen expand.
3. Exhale slowly, feeling your abdomen contract.
4. Repeat this process, focusing on the slow, deliberate pace of each breath.

Regular practice of deep diaphragmatic breathing enhances body awareness and can lead to a calmer, more centered state, helping you manage anxiety and improve emotional well-being.

Box Breathing

Box breathing is a structured technique that involves equal timing for inhaling, holding, exhaling, and pausing. This method is particularly useful for beginners and can be easily adapted to various situations, like stressful meetings and moments of anxiety.

HOW TO PRACTICE

1. Inhale through your nose for a count of four.
2. Hold your breath at the top for a count of four.
3. Exhale slowly through your mouth for a count of four.
4. Hold your breath out for a final count of four.
5. Repeat the sequence several times.

Imagine you're about to give a presentation, and you're feeling nervous. Instead of letting the anxiety take over, you decide to use box breathing to calm your mind and focus.

You take a moment to sit quietly and start by inhaling deeply through your nose for a count of four. You then hold your breath for a count of four, allowing yourself to feel centered. Slowly, you exhale through your mouth for a count of four, releasing any tension. Finally, you hold your breath out for another count of four.

After repeating this sequence a few times, you notice your heart rate slows, and you feel more grounded. Your mind is clearer, and you're better prepared to face the presentation with a calm and focused mindset. Box breathing has helped you regain control over your stress, turning a potentially overwhelming moment into an opportunity for calm and clarity.

Sighing Breath

An effective method for alleviating accumulated stress in just a few deep breaths.

HOW TO PRACTICE

1. Take a deep breath in through your nose.
2. Exhale with an audible sigh.
3. Repeat three to four times, allowing your body to relax.

Resonant Breathing

This technique helps synchronize breathing with the heart rate, creating a calming effect.

HOW TO PRACTICE

1. Inhale for five to six seconds.
2. Exhale for five to six seconds.
3. Keep the breath steady and rhythmic for 5–10 minutes.

Humming Bee Breath

This technique uses sound vibrations to soothe the nervous system and quiet the mind.

HOW TO PRACTICE

1. Inhale deeply through your nose.
2. Exhale while making a soft humming "mmm" sound.
3. Feel the vibration in your head and chest.
4. Repeat 5–10 times.

The 5-4-3-2-1 Technique

This technique enhances mindfulness through sensory awareness, helping to redirect your attention away from stressors and bring you back to the present moment. It encourages you to engage with your environment, calming your mind by focusing on sensory input.

HOW TO PRACTICE

1. Identify five things you can see around you.
2. Notice four things you can touch.
3. Acknowledge three sounds you can hear.
4. Recognize two scents you can smell.
5. Identify one thing you can taste.
6. Pair this with slow, controlled breaths, grounding you in the present.

The 5-4-3-2-1 technique is a simple mindfulness practice that grounds you in the present by engaging your senses. It effectively shifts focus from stress and anxiety, allowing for a calming reconnection with your surroundings.

Imagine you're in the middle of a high-pressure workday. You have back-to-back meetings, a looming deadline, and an inbox overflowing with emails. Feeling overwhelmed, you decide to take a moment to practice the 5-4-3-2-1 technique at your desk.

1. Identify five things you can see around you.
- ☐ The blue sticky notes on your monitor.
- ☐ The coffee mug that is half full.
- ☐ A potted plant sitting on the corner of your desk.
- ☐ Your coworker's colorful water bottle on the neighboring desk.
- ☐ The clock on the wall showing the time.

2. Notice four things you can touch.

- ☐ The smooth surface of your desk.
- ☐ The warmth of your coffee mug.
- ☐ The fabric of your chair.
- ☐ The keys of your keyboard.

3. Acknowledge three sounds you can hear.

- ☐ The quiet hum of the air-conditioning.
- ☐ The soft tapping of keyboards nearby.
- ☐ The muffled sound of voices from a distant meeting room.

4. Recognize two scents you can smell.

- ☐ The smell of coffee that has been freshly brewed.
- ☐ The hand sanitizer that you applied earlier in the day.

5. Identify one thing you can taste.

- ☐ Take a sip of your coffee and notice its taste.

6. Pair this with slow, controlled breaths, grounding you in the present.

As you move through each step, you pair the exercise with slow, deep breaths, inhaling deeply through your nose and exhaling slowly through your mouth. By the end of the practice, you feel calmer and more focused, ready to tackle the next task on your to-do list.

Lion's Breath

This is a dynamic breathing technique that helps release tension and increase energy. It helps to make one's body feel energized and relieve tension in the jaw muscles.

HOW TO PRACTICE

1. Find a comfortable seated position, either resting on your heels or crossing your legs.
2. Place your palms firmly on your knees with your fingers spread apart.
3. Take a deep breath in through your nose and open your eyes as wide as possible.
4. Simultaneously, open your mouth fully and extend your tongue, directing the tip toward your chin.
5. Tighten the muscles at the front of your throat while exhaling through your mouth, producing a prolonged "haaa" sound.
6. Focus your gaze on the area between your eyebrows or the tip of your nose.
7. Repeat this breathing exercise two to three times.

Regular practice of Lion's Breath can enhance your energy and mental clarity. This dynamic technique boosts energy circulation while promoting relaxation, equipping you to tackle daily challenges with your newfound energy.

MEDITATION RESOURCE

Mindful Moments

Feeling overwhelmed, anxious, or rushing through life? *Mindful Moments* is your pause button. Hosted by Dr. Jerome Puryear, each short, guided meditation helps you slow down, breathe deeply, and reconnect with yourself—anytime, anywhere.

In just 10 minutes, you'll explore practices for releasing anger, easing emotional pain, building self-confidence, and embracing stillness. These sessions aren't just a break from your day—they're a tool for lasting calm, clarity, and compassion.

Perfect for beginners building a meditation habit or seasoned practitioners looking for a quick reset, *Mindful Moments* offers simple, effective techniques to nurture your lifelong wellness. Join us in finding peace in the middle of your busy days. Follow *Mindful Moments* and take your first step toward a calmer, more centered life—one breath at a time.

Scan the QR codes below or search for *Mindful Moments* by Dr. Jerome Puryear to listen to the meditation playlist on Spotify or YouTube.

SPOTIFY   YOUTUBE

Acknowledgments

This book represents the culmination of both personal and professional experiences, which have profoundly shaped my journey of understanding how to release past pain and trauma, and to embrace the freedom of new beginnings. The process of composing these pages has been both a healing endeavor and a distinct privilege, and I am deeply honored to extend this message to adolescents, parents, educators, and healers who may discover strength and encouragement within these words.

I extend my deepest gratitude to my parents, whose unwavering love and foundational values instilled within me a spirit of resilience, and to my sisters, whose presence has consistently served as a source of comfort and inspiration. To my children, who perpetually remind me of the inherent beauty in growth, change, and unconditional love—you are my most profound educators. I am equally thankful for the support of my close friends and for the numerous individuals who have intersected with my path, each imparting invaluable lessons and encouragement that have facilitated my personal development.

This book would not have been realized without the collective wisdom, steadfast support, and profound kindness of all those who believed in my vision and inspired me to persevere. Your unwavering faith has been instrumental in fueling my passion to disseminate this message of healing and hope to others.

From the depths of my heart, I am genuinely and eternally grateful.

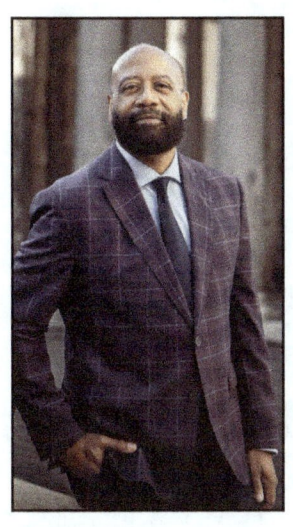

Dr. Jerome Puryear, MD, MBA, Dipl ABOM, is a physician, entrepreneur, and wellness advocate with over 25 years of experience helping people break free from stress, anxiety, and self-doubt. Drawing on his unique blend of medical expertise, business insight, and certification as a Duke-trained Health & Well-Being Coach, he empowers teens and young adults to release emotional burdens and live with greater clarity, resilience, and purpose. *Mastering the Art of Letting Go of Emotional Pain & Toxic Relationships* is his guide to building a healthier, more authentic life—starting from the inside out.

THANK YOU FOR READING

Your journey means so much.

If this book gave you hope, helped you let go,
or reminded you of your own strength,
I'd love to hear from you.

Please take a moment to leave a review on Amazon—
your words help this message reach others who need it too.

Scan the QR code below
to share your thoughts.

Your reflection might be exactly
what someone else needs
to start their healing journey.